Attitudes on Voting in 2020

Preparing for Elections During a Pandemic

JENNIFER KAVANAGH, C. BEN GIBSON, QUENTIN E. HODGSON

RAND CORPORATION

For more information on this publication, visit **www.rand.org/t/RRA112-9**

Library of Congress Cataloging-in-Publication Data is available for this publication.
ISBN: 978-1-9774-0564-7

Published by the RAND Corporation, Santa Monica, Calif.

Cover image: Adobe Stock/rawpixel.com

Preface

In this report, we consider the perceptions of 2,389 survey respondents about the safety and integrity of elections in November 2020 and about the preparedness of local officials to manage elections in the pandemic context. We consider which populations are more or less likely to have confidence in the physical safety of the November elections, the accurate counting of votes, and the preparation of local officials to conduct an election given the likelihood of continuing pandemic conditions through the rest of 2020. We also explore how perceptions are related to intention to vote and whether there is evidence of a decline in intention to vote compared with 2016 that might be associated with the challenges and risks of the pandemic. The data used in this report come from a RAND Corporation American Life Panel survey conducted in May and June 2020.

This report is part of RAND's Countering Truth Decay initiative, which is focused on restoring the role of facts, data, and analysis in U.S. political and civil discourse and the policymaking process. The original report, *Truth Decay: An Initial Exploration of the Diminishing Role of Facts and Analysis in American Public Life*,[1] laid out a research agenda for studying and developing solutions to the Truth Decay challenge. Truth Decay worsens when individuals lose trust in institutions that could serve as sources of factual information. Legitimate and safe elections can be a first step toward building and maintaining a govern-

[1] Jennifer Kavanagh and Michael D. Rich, *Truth Decay: An Initial Exploration of the Diminishing Role of Facts and Analysis in American Public Life*, Santa Monica, Calif.: RAND Corporation, RR-2314-RC, 2018.

ment that people trust. This report considers public perceptions of the safety and integrity of elections in pandemic conditions and views of local preparedness for the elections.

Funding

Funding for RAND's Countering Truth Decay research initiative is provided by gifts from RAND supporters and income from operations. RAND would like to recognize the Joel and Joanne Mogy Truth Decay Fellowship, established by the Mogys in 2020 to support research on Truth Decay, civics, and democracy. The authors drew from the Mogys' generous gift to fund this project.

Contents

Boxes, Figures, and Tables

Boxes

Figures

Tables

Summary

In this report, we consider the attitudes of 2,389 survey respondents about the safety and integrity of elections in November 2020 and about the preparedness of local officials to manage elections in the coronavirus disease 2019 (COVID-19) pandemic context. We also explore how these perceptions are related to intention to vote. The data come from a RAND Corporation American Life Panel survey conducted in May and June 2020.

This report addresses two key issues:

- First, we consider respondent perceptions of safety, election integrity, and preparedness. Specifically, we are interested in understanding (1) which populations are most likely to have concerns about the safety and integrity of the 2020 election and about the preparedness of local officials to execute these elections and (2) which populations expect the election to be safe, votes to be counted accurately, and officials to be prepared. Given that few elections have been conducted under pandemic conditions in U.S. history, these analyses will provide a unique baseline, which is useful in its own right and as a comparison for future analyses.
- Second, we consider intention to vote within the pandemic context. We look at how perceptions of safety, election integrity, and preparedness shape intention to vote among respondents who plan to vote. We consider how our analysis compares with past work on factors that drive intention to vote. We also compare intentions in 2020 with those in 2016 to explore whether there seem to be large shifts that might be attributable to the pandemic. These analyses can inform an understanding of how (and how

significantly) the ongoing pandemic might influence intention to vote. Although past work has considered the effects of security threats and political violence on election turnout, there is limited analysis of how public health emergencies might influence intention to vote. This analysis provides a fresh look at this question from the perspective of the pandemic.

This report provides a snapshot of U.S. attitudes and intentions regarding the November 2020 election given the COVID-19 pandemic. It also provides some insight into how, given the pandemic context, attitudes about the safety and integrity of the 2020 election could shape intention to vote and how this might vary across demographic groups. The report will be useful for stakeholders seeking to ensure that pandemic-related concerns do not deter voters who would otherwise participate in the November 2020 election, and it can help inform messaging and communication strategies around election preparations for election officials seeking to mitigate voter uncertainties about the November 2020 election.

Perceptions of Safety, Election Integrity, and Preparedness

A majority of respondents said that they expect that the 2020 election will be physically safe from COVID-19 health risks, that their votes will be counted accurately despite the challenges of the pandemic, and that local officials are prepared to carry out elections successfully despite the additional challenges. However, about one-third of respondents reported a lack of certainty across all three dimensions. Furthermore, we found that respondents who said that they do not expect elections to be physically safe were also more likely to question whether their vote will be counted accurately and whether officials will be prepared.

Our analysis also highlights some relevant cross-group differences in perceptions that might be relevant to the crafting and dissemination of strategic messages about mitigations and preparations for use by election officials:

- Self-identified Republicans are more likely than self-identified Democrats to expect elections to be safe and election officials to be prepared, but Republicans express somewhat more concern than Democrats do about integrity (their votes being counted accurately) under pandemic conditions.
- All else being equal, older voters had higher perceptions of safety and preparedness and more confidence in election integrity than did younger voters.
- Race and ethnicity were also relevant. We found that Black and Hispanic respondents tended to be less likely than White and non-Hispanic respondents to expect their votes to be counted accurately, given the pandemic context. Hispanic respondents were also less likely than non-Hispanic respondents to report confidence in the preparedness of local officials. Differences in perception of safety along racial lines were considerably smaller.

Risk Mitigations

We also considered respondent attitudes toward three possible mitigations that could reduce the public health risk: sanitation and social distancing at poll locations, distribution of mail-in ballots to all registered voters, and online voting. We found widespread support for sanitation and social distancing at poll locations but lower support for sending mail-in ballots to all registered voters or using online voting. Our analysis showed that many of the same factors that influence perceptions about future conditions also affect attitudes toward various mitigations. We observed that self-identified Republicans are more likely to support sanitation and social distancing at the polls but less likely to support expanded distribution of mail-in ballots to all registered voters and online voting. Education also matters; respondents who reported higher levels of education tended to be more supportive than respondents with lower levels of education of social distancing and sanitation at the polls and of expanded distribution of mail-in ballots to all registered voters as mitigation strategies for pandemic-related risks. Respondents living in urban areas expressed higher support than did rural respondents for both sending mail-in ballots to all registered voters and voting online. Finally, Hispanic and Black respondents were less supportive than non-Hispanic and White respondents, respectively, were about sending mail-in ballots to all registered voters; Hispanic respondents did, however, express more support than non-Hispanic respondents for online voting.

Perceptions and Intention to Vote

We also consider how perceptions of safety, election integrity, and preparedness are associated with intention to vote. In the aggregate, we found little evidence that intention to vote is significantly lower among our group of respondents than was the case at a similar point in 2016 for these same respondents. We found only a small number of respondents who participated in both a 2016 survey and our 2020 survey who reported large changes in their intention to vote. We also found a notable increase in the proportion of respondents planning to vote by mail rather than in person compared with self-reported voting methods in past elections. Many respondents seem to be making plans to vote using remote methods (where available); few seemed to be deciding not to vote.

However, we did find that perceived safety has a positive relationship with intention to vote—voters who expect elections to be safe express higher intention to vote than those who do not. We found little independent relationship between intention to vote and perceptions of integrity and preparedness, but we did observe that safety and integrity matter more to intention to vote for some voters than others. For example, Black respondents seemed less influenced by perception of safety than White respondents. Respondents with higher levels of education similarly appeared to be less strongly influenced by their assessments of integrity than those who reported having lower levels of education. Because these perceptions of safety, election integrity, and preparedness seem to be related to each other, it is possible that individuals whose safety concerns reduce their intention to vote might also have concerns about integrity and preparedness that further depress their intention to vote.

Implications

The analyses in this report yield several useful observations for policymakers and election officials as they plan for the November 2020 election.

Intention to Vote Seems Robust to Pandemic Concerns

Although there is some evidence that safety concerns are associated with lower intention to vote, there is little evidence that voters are significantly less likely to vote in this pandemic context than they were in 2016. This is reassuring for those concerned that the pandemic would depress turnout, but we note that at least some portion of the stability in voters' intention to vote might reflect their expectations about steps that local officials will take to mitigate risk. Failure to take those steps and communicate with the public about ongoing preparations could result in a different outcome.

Ensuring and Messaging a Commitment to Both Safety and Integrity Will Be Important

Our analyses indicate that perception of safety is more strongly related to intention to vote, but that perception of integrity also matters to some groups. Election integrity is a key concern in all elections and can encompass everything from protecting against cyber threats and voter fraud to ensuring voter privacy, but the pandemic context will bring additional logistical challenges, especially in places where the volume of mail-in ballots is expected to be significantly greater than usual (straining available resources) or where staffing sufficient polling places will make in-person voting more difficult. Election officials interested in ensuring that those who would otherwise vote are not deterred from doing so in 2020 because of pandemic-related concerns should prioritize safety and election integrity equally and clearly communicate with constituents about the steps being taken. This could mean additional investments in equipment or larger efforts to recruit additional pollworkers or acquire protective gear for pollworkers.

Offering No-Excuse Mail-In Options Could Mitigate Safety Concerns

We found that voters who live in Western states that offer mail-in options with no excuse required (hereafter referred to as *no-excuse mail-in*) were more likely to report that they expected the 2020 general election to be free from health-related risks. We also observed that respondents who did not report an expectation that the 2020 election would be free from health concerns were more likely to report an intention to switch to mail-in voting. We cannot make causal arguments, but this result at least suggests that states interested in mitigating the safety concerns of voters should consider offering a no-excuse mail-in option if one does not already exist. It is worth noting that only 16 states do not have such an option—and several of these states have implemented no-excuse provisions for 2020. Choosing to shift to a no-excuse mail-in system does have implications for access and integrity (both outside the scope of this report), and states must also consider current laws and logistical considerations before pursuing such a change. There will not be one approach that works everywhere, but our analysis can be one factor among many informing policymaker choices.

Messaging Targeted at Groups That Question Safety, Integrity, and Preparedness Might Be Most Efficient at Mitigating Voter Concerns

Our analyses clearly showed that different groups have different perceptions of safety, election integrity, and preparedness of local officials for the 2020 election and that the relationship between perceptions and intention to vote similarly varies across demographic groups. Although election officials and policymakers might wish to communicate broadly about their preparations for the 2020 election, our analyses suggest that such a campaign's effects would be maximized by targeting these messages at specific groups that seem most prone to such concerns. First, younger voters seem to have more concerns than do older voters, but older respondents appear to be more influenced by any negative perceptions when deciding whether to vote. In this case, messages might need to be developed for each audience. Second, minority groups appear more likely to have concerns about safety, election integrity, and preparedness. Notably, young and minority voters tend to have lower turnout rates generally than older and nonminority voters. For policymakers interested in ensuring that the pandemic does not drive further disparities in this area, communication targeted at these groups could be a useful tool. Finally, we note that Republican and Democratic respondents appeared to differ in their perceptions of risk: Republicans expressed more concern about election integrity; Democrats expressed more concern about safety. This reaffirms the notion that any communication strategy must equally emphasize both dimensions.

Final Thoughts

Efforts to understand how voters perceive the public health and election integrity risks stemming from the pandemic and how such risks might affect voting behavior will be ongoing between now and the November elections. The trajectory of the pandemic, individual risk tolerance, mitigation strategies and messaging campaigns by election officials, and the changing political and social context are all likely to inform individuals' perceptions and intention to vote.

This report provides a baseline for exploring the evolution of these attitudes over the next several months, and the insights provided herein can inform policymakers and election officials who have an interest in mitigating voter safety and integrity concerns. However, a few caveats—also noted elsewhere in the report—are worth discussing here. First, when assessing expectations about safety and integrity, we cannot determine the extent to which an individual's response is based on assumptions about mitigations that public officials will take or about the trajectory of the virus. If such assumptions are factored in, then individual expectations might look very different. Second, when comparing intention to vote among 2016 respondents with that of 2020 respondents, we can only say that, in general, we saw no dramatic change. We cannot directly attribute this to a lack of response to the pandemic because any individual's decision to vote is based on myriad considerations.

Finally, our survey results—and, by extension, the results of our analysis—are likely influenced by the point in time at which the survey was conducted. Late May and early June was a period during which the most-severe effects of the pandemic had been felt in the Northeast and mid-Atlantic region, when the majority of states in this region turned the corner and were approaching reopening. Two months later, the picture already looks different, with the virus having surged in the South and the West and with some states reinstituting restrictions. All this could have shifted some public attitudes in these states. It will be important to continue to track voter attitudes through the fall about the 2020 general election, their perceptions of safety and integrity, and their intention to vote.

Acknowledgments

We appreciate the support of Michael Rich, Terrence Kelly, Henry Willis, Jordan Fischbach, Katherine Carman, Sangita Baxi, Erica Robles, and Steph Bingley. We are also grateful for feedback from our reviewers: Scott Bates, Christopher Deluzio, Melissa Finucane, Brian Jenkins, Juliette Kayyem, Geoffrey McGovern, Andrew Parker, Michael Pollard, and James Thomson. Their contributions significantly improved the report. We thank Arwen Bicknell for her expert editorial assistance on this report.

CHAPTER ONE

Introduction

The ongoing coronavirus disease 2019 (COVID-19) pandemic presents a set of new challenges to state and local election officials as they plan for the November 2020 general election. First, there are public health considerations. In-person voting poses an increased risk of virus spread by assembling large groups of people in common spaces and by shared use of common equipment. Social distancing, sanitation, and enforcement of mask-wearing are possible mitigations, but all require investment to implement. Second, there are logistical considerations. In-person voting creates issues not only of sanitation but also of staffing. Primary elections in some states were hindered as officials struggled to fully staff polling locations because of pollworker reluctance to risk exposure to the virus.[1] For mail-in voting, election officials will likely have to deal with an increase in mail-in ballots (if the number of primary returns are any indication) and the challenges of accurately processing, counting, and verifying these ballots.[2] States are likely to vary in their response to these challenges; responses will depend on local conditions, existing election law, and the attitudes of elected officials at the state level toward issues of access and election integrity.[3]

---

[1] For example, see Alexa Ura, "Two Major Texas Counties Are Trimming Polling Locations as Workers Pull Out over Coronavirus," *Texas Tribune*, July 9, 2020.

[2] For example, see Charles Stewart III, "Election Updates: Mail Ballot Watch," MIT Election Data and Science Lab, July 6, 2020.

[3] The companion reports to this one provide additional details on state election laws and processes and the safety, access, integrity, and logistical considerations associated with different election procedures and requirements. See, respectively, Jennifer Kavanagh,

States with existing universal mail-in voting, for instance, will not need to make many changes. Officials in states where the spread of the COVID-19 virus is limited might feel confident in making few modifications to existing plans. State legislatures and state executives have demonstrated varying responses to the COVID-19 crisis and have expressed varying attitudes about remote versus in-person voting, all of which are likely to shape decisions about how best to execute an election in the pandemic context.[4]

Another important consideration for policymakers as they develop plans for the November 2020 election is how eligible voters perceive the health risks of voting during a pandemic, the risks to election integrity or security that might result from the pandemic, and the preparation of local officials. Election officials might wish to consider public attitudes and perceptions in their decisions about election processes and in their messaging about the election itself. For example, election officials who perceive public concerns about the safety of in-person voting might wish to counter those concerns by ensuring that remote options are available or by messaging information about alternative voting methods or the safety measures being taken at the polling locations.[5]

To inform policymaker decisions and messaging around the November 2020 election, we used a survey of 2,389 Americans through RAND's American Life Panel,[6] asking the following ques-

---

Quentin E. Hodgson, C. Ben Gibson, and Samantha Cherney, *An Assessment of State Voting Processes: Preparing for Elections During a Pandemic*, Santa Monica, Calif.: RAND Corporation, RR-A112-8, 2020; and Quentin E. Hodgson, Jennifer Kavanagh, Anusree Garg, Edward W. Chan, and Christine Sovak, *Options for Ensuring Safe Elections: Preparing for Elections During a Pandemic*, Santa Monica, Calif.: RAND Corporation, RR-A112-10, 2020.

[4] For more on state differences in terms of preparation for conducting elections in the pandemic context, see Kavanagh et al., 2020.

[5] Of course, there also might be stakeholders who benefit from public health concerns that keep people away from the polls and who might interfere with efforts to alleviate public concerns. The discussion and recommendations in this report are aimed primarily at stakeholders who seek to ensure that election safety, access, and integrity are not diminished by the COVID-19 pandemic.

[6] The American Life Panel is a nationally representative, probability-based, longitudinal survey maintained by the RAND Corporation with about 3,000 active participants. The sample is internet-based, and respondents who do not have access to needed technology are

tions about intention to vote, the methods by which they expect to vote, how physically safe and secure they expect the fall election to be, and what actions states should take to ensure the safety and legitimacy of elections. Specifically, we asked:

- When was the last time you voted? How did you cast your ballot?
- How likely are you to vote in the November 2020 election and how will you cast your ballot?
- Do you believe that voting in November 2020 will be physically safe, given the ongoing pandemic?
- Do you believe that your vote will be counted accurately in November 2020, given the ongoing pandemic?
- Do you think local officials are prepared to safeguard your physical health from risks associated with COVID-19 during the 2020 presidential election?
- What steps should local officials take to ensure safe elections in 2020?[7]

We use the responses to these questions to consider two key issues:

- First, we consider respondent perceptions of safety, election integrity, and preparedness. Specifically, we are interested in understanding (1) which populations are most likely to have concerns about the safety and integrity of the 2020 election and about the preparedness of local officials to execute these elections, and (2) which populations expect the election to be safe, votes to be counted accurately, and officials to be prepared. Few elections have been conducted under pandemic conditions in U.S. history, so these analyses will provide a unique baseline, which is useful in its own right and as a comparison for future analyses.

---

provided a tablet and internet access. Completion of surveys is voluntary and respondents are remunerated for their time. For more information, see RAND Corporation, "RAND American Life Panel," webpage, undated.

[7] These questions summarize the topics covered in the survey. For exact wording, see the appendix. For respondents who indicated that they would not vote, we asked them about their perceptions of whether other people would be safe.

- Second, we consider intention to vote within the pandemic context. We look at how perceptions of safety, election integrity, and preparedness shape intention to vote for those who do plan to vote. We consider how our analysis compares with past work on factors that drive intention to vote, and we compare intention to vote among voters in 2020 with that of voters in 2016 to explore whether there seem to be large shifts that might be attributable to the pandemic. These analyses can inform an understanding of how (and how significantly) the ongoing pandemic might influence intention to vote. Although past work has considered the effects of security threats and political violence on election turnout, there is limited analysis of how public health emergencies influence intention to vote. This analysis provides a fresh look at this question from the perspective of the COVID-19 pandemic.

This report provides a snapshot of U.S. attitudes regarding the November 2020 election, and it provides some insight into how, given the pandemic context, attitudes about the safety and integrity of the 2020 election might shape intentions to vote (and how these attitudes and intentions might vary across demographic groups). We use the results to make recommendations for policymakers and election officials about pre-election messaging to counter voter concerns. These recommendations will be useful for stakeholders seeking to ensure that pandemic-related concerns do not deter voters who would otherwise participate in the November 2020 election. They can also inform messaging and communication strategies around preparations for election officials seeking to mitigate voter uncertainties about the November 2020 election.

CHAPTER TWO

Assessments of Safety, Integrity, and Preparedness

The first questions we considered were how voters perceive the physical safety of the election from a public health perspective, the integrity of election processes (whether they thought their own vote would be counted accurately, given the pandemic context), and the preparedness of their local officials to conduct the November 2020 election. Although there is extensive research on such topics as election security, integrity, and administration, little of it pertains to a pandemic context, partly because the pandemic itself is a novel event.

Understanding which groups of eligible voters might be more or less concerned about safety, about whether their vote will count, and about the preparedness of local election officials can inform both strategies to mitigate voter concerns and methods of communicating those mitigation strategies. We explore the relationships among various demographic, geographic, and attitudinal factors that might be associated with perceptions of safety, election integrity, and preparedness. We chose factors that seem likely to shape individual risk tolerance, political attitudes, and trust in institutions. Table 2.1 lists the full set of variables considered. As we present the results, we report only those that we found to have a statistically significant relationship with individual perceptions. Our analyses are weighted to account for ways in which our sample differs from the general population. In particular, we used weights that account for partisanship and vote history to bal-

Table 2.1
Variables Featured in Perception Models

Variable	Definition
Age	Divided into ranges (e.g., 24–30, 31–40, 41–50, etc.)
Gender	Male, female
Race	White/Caucasian, American Indian, Asian/Pacific Islander, Black/African American, other
Hispanic ethnicity	Yes, no
Education	Level of schooling completed (less than college, college degree, postgraduate degree)
Political party preference	Democrat, Republican, independent, other, unsure
Voted in 2016 and/or 2018	Individual reported voting most recently either in 2016 or 2018
Reported voting method in most recent election	Method used to vote in most recent election (in-person, mail-in, etc.)
Residence location	Urban or rural status
No-excuse mail-in voting state	Lives in a state with no-excuse mail-in voting option
Region	Midwest, Northeast, South, West
Perception of safety	Response to: Do you feel that you will be safe from risks to your physical health stemming from COVID-19?
Perception of integrity	Response to: Do you feel that your vote will be counted accurately in light of the current pandemic?
Perception of preparedness	Response to: Do you believe local elections officials are prepared to safeguard your physical health from risks associated with COVID-19 during the 2020 presidential election?

NOTE: We also used several interaction terms intended to explore interactions between perceptions. However, the model with interactions did not yield significantly different results than the simpler models. For more details, see the appendix.

ance the fact that nonvoters might be underrepresented among respondents.[1] We provide detailed results in the appendix.

Assessments of Safety

First, we asked respondents *"When you think about voting in November 2020, do you feel that you will be safe from risks to your physical health stemming from COVID-19?"* (we call this *perception of safety*). Respondents were given three choices: yes, no, or unsure. We found that about 60 percent of those who expected to vote responded that they would feel safe, 15 percent said that they would not, and the other 25 percent reported that they were uncertain.[2] In interpreting these results, it is worth noting that we cannot fully disentangle those who reported that they would feel safe if the election were held under the status quo, with no change in virus prevalence and without any mitigations to counter health risks, from those who expect that they will feel safe in November, given their assumptions about mitigations that will be implemented or progress in containing the virus. In other words, there might be respondents who responded "yes" to this question only on the basis of their assumptions.[3] Although this is a limitation, we addressed this concern somewhat by asking later in the survey about respondent attitudes toward possible mitigations. These responses at least provide insight into the types of mitigations that individual respondents might have been thinking about. We discuss these results at the end of this chapter.

We used statistical analysis to understand which demographic, attitudinal, and geographic characteristics are most relevant to the

---

[1] For methodological details on these weights, see Michael S. Pollard and Joshua Mendelsohn, *Methodology of the 2016 RAND Presidential Election Panel Survey (PEPS)*, RAND Corporation, RR-1460-RC/UCLA, 2016 (our data comes from wave 3). For more on the underrepresentation of nonvoters in surveys, see John O. Brehm, *The Phantom Respondents: Opinion Surveys and Political Representation*, Ann Arbor: University of Michigan Press, 2009.

[2] This analysis uses the weights previously described.

[3] Similar assumptions might affect how voters respond to questions about integrity and preparedness.

safety risk perceptions of respondents.[4] We categorized voters into two groups: those who responded "yes" (we label these individuals as certain about the safety of the election) and those who responded "no" or "unsure" (we label these individuals as uncertain). We used several different respondent individual characteristics, such as age, race, gender, education, political party preference, and region of residence.[5] Box 2.1 summarizes which specific variables appear statistically significant and the direction of their relationship with perceptions of safety. The full results and details on our methodology are provided in the appendix.

Of all characteristics, partisanship is the largest and most significant predictor of expectations about election safety. Republicans were significantly more likely to expect that the upcoming election would be free of physical health risks than their Democratic or independent counterparts. Independent of other characteristics, we estimate that self-identified Republicans were about 1.5 times more likely than Democrats to express certainty in the safety of the 2020 election from a personal health perspective. In the current political climate, and given existing data on public concern about COVID-19 generally (which have shown greater concern among Democrats), it is not surprising that political party preference is associated with perceptions of safety in this way.[6] Voting history also matters. Those respondents who reported having voted in 2016 or 2018 were significantly more likely to report that they expected the 2020 election to be safe.

We found a few relevant demographic characteristics that are associated with perception of safety, but perhaps fewer than might be expected. First, age matters, but this can largely be explained by differences in partisanship and race across age groups. Respondents under 30 years of age seemed most likely to report uncertainty about physical

---

[4] Specifically, we used logistic regression. Our method is described in more detail in the appendix.

[5] Details of our analysis, including full regression results, are provided in the appendix.

[6] For example, see Pew Research Center, "Republicans, Democrats Move Even Further Apart in Coronavirus Concerns," June 25, 2020. These differences could result from any number of factors, such as cross-party differences in trust in institutions or elite cues. David Darmofal, "Elite Cues and Citizen Disagreement with Expert Opinion," *Political Research Quarterly*, Vol. 58, No. 3, 2005.

BOX 2.1

Demographic and Geographic Factors Associated with Perception of Safety

Characteristics associated with perception of safety:

- age***
- Republican, independent (compared with Democrat)***
- male (compared with female)*
- expect vote to be counted***
- voted in 2016 and/or 2018***
- believe local officials are prepared***
- live in the West (compared with Northeast)**

Characteristics associated with uncertainty about safety:

- Hispanic*

* $p < 0.05$ (moderate statistical significance); ** $p < 0.01$ (high statistical significance); *** $p < 0.001$ (very high statistical significance).
NOTES: Survey question was phrased as "When you think about voting in November 2020, do you feel that you will be safe from risks to your physical health stemming from COVID-19?" These models are unweighted but results from weighted models were substantively the same. As a robustness check, we also ran models that exclude the other perception variables (e.g., looking at perception of safety without including perceptions of integrity or preparedness). We found the results mostly unchanged. For details, see the appendix.

safety, despite being at lower risk of mortality from the disease.[7] However, once controls for political party affiliation and race were added, older respondents reported similar levels of uncertainty. Considered on its own, race or ethnicity plays only a small role in perceptions of safety. Respondents of Hispanic ethnicity were less likely than non-Hispanic respondents to report that they expect the election to be safe.

7 Smriti Mallapaty, "How Deadly Is the Coronavirus? Scientists Are Close to an Answer," *Nature*, Vol. 582, June 16, 2020, pp. 467–468.

We also found geographic differences in perceptions of safety. Voters in the West were more likely than voters in the Northeast to report that they expect physical safety at the polls in November. It is possible that this reflects different regional experiences with COVID-19 (in terms of the number of cases and deaths) at the time of the survey in late May and June 2020. It is possible that we might see a different set of regional relationships as the number of cases rises in the West and the South or no difference at all if experiences and perceptions become more equal. Consistent with our assessment that local conditions might matter, voters who perceive local officials to be well prepared to safeguard public health during the election (*perception of preparedness*) and those who are certain that their vote will be counted accurately (*perception of integrity*) (both also taken from our survey) are also more likely to report feelings of personal safety.

Using the results of this statistical analysis, we next consider how perceptions of safety differ based on characteristics identified as statistically significant. This analysis is useful because it allows us to observe how much the characteristics identified in Table 2.1 appear to matter when considering perceptions that the November 2020 election will be safe from health risks. Figure 2.1 illustrates predicted probabilities, which are the statistical model's predictions about how the average person who matches the group of interest would respond to the question about the safety of the 2020 election (that is, how likely this average person is to respond yes or no/unsure). For example, a comparison between those who reported voting in 2016 and/or 2018 and those who did not assesses the average respondent in each group; the assessment would therefore incorporate the fact that frequent voters tend to be older than infrequent voters and that minority groups tend to turn out at lower rates than nonminority voters. As another example, the comparison of predicted probabilities between Republicans and Democrats considers the average respondent in each group and therefore will incorporate differences in age, race, and region of residence. All variables shown in Figure 2.1 were found to have independent effects above and beyond other characteristics (that is, they are identified in the statistical model as being statistically significant).

Figure 2.1
Predicted Percentage of Agreement with Perception of Safety Survey Question

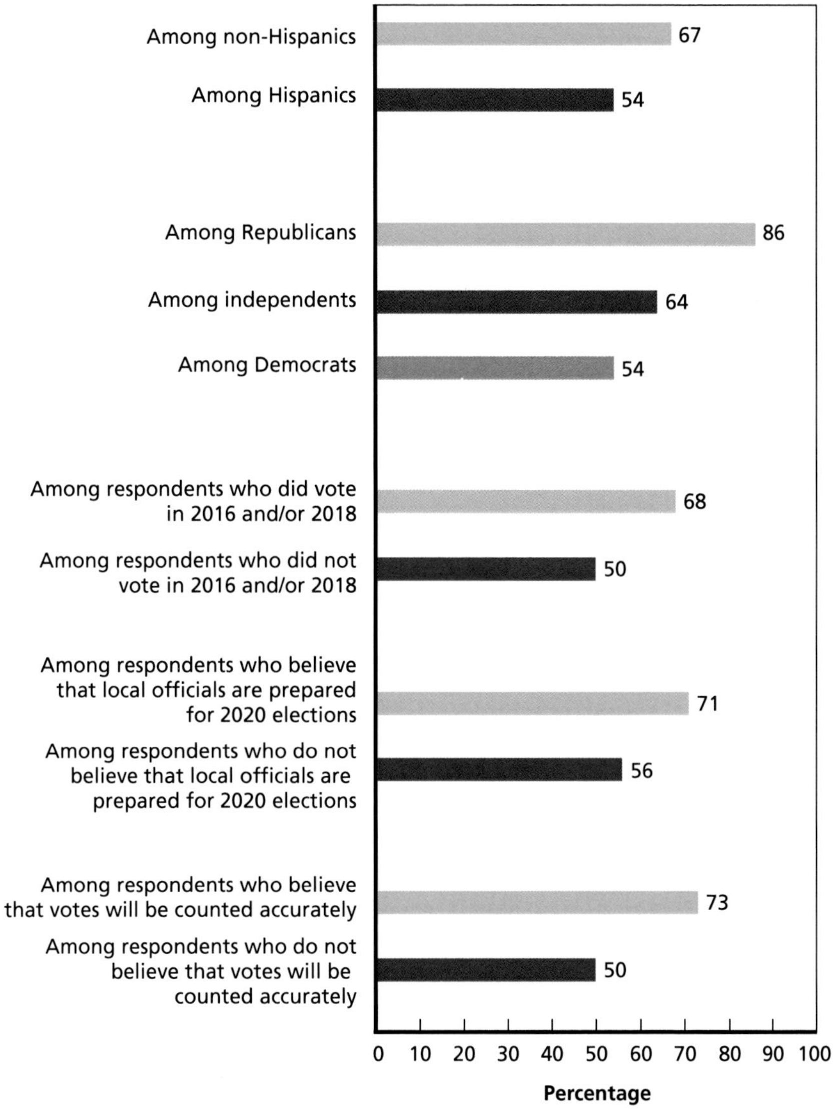

NOTE: Predicted probabilities use population weights. The survey question phrasing was "When you think about voting in November 2020, do you feel that you will be safe from risks to your physical health stemming from COVID-19?"

Figure 2.1 shows that partisanship is one of the most significant factors. According to the model, we would expect that, among Republicans, about 86 percent would report that they expect the November election to be safe, while only 54 percent among Democrats would report the same, and this difference is significant after accounting for other characteristics. Similarly, respondents who voted in 2016 or 2018 are predicted to be more likely to report that they expect the election to be safe (68 percent) than those who did not report voting in 2016 and/or 2018 (50 percent). Those who reported Hispanic ethnicity are predicted to be less likely to expect that the election will be safe (54 percent) than those who did not report Hispanic ethnicity (67 percent).

Several other relationships are worth noting:

- Those who have concerns about election integrity are considerably more likely than those who do not to report uncertainty about safety (73 percent versus 50 percent).
- Those who are certain about the preparedness of local officials are predicted to be more certain about safety than those who have less-positive assessments of preparedness (71 percent versus 56 percent). This suggests that at least some portion of perceptions of safety might be influenced by respondent expectations about steps that their local officials will take to mitigate health risks.

The substantive effect of other variables on perceptions of safety appears smaller.

Assessments of Election Integrity

Next, we asked respondents *"Do you feel that your vote will be counted accurately in light of the current pandemic?"* (we call this *perception of integrity*).[8] Respondents were given three choices: yes, no, and unsure.

---

[8] Other forms of election integrity, such as potential for voter fraud or cyber threats to election systems, are not addressed.

About 55 percent of voters expressed confidence that their vote would be counted accurately; 7 percent said that their vote would not be counted accurately; and 38 percent responded that they were not certain. This level of uncertainty is notable because it suggests that more than one-third of respondents expressed some level of doubt about whether a secure and accurate election can be carried out while the COVID-19 crisis persists. Of course, it is important to note that although we did ask about perceptions "in light of the current pandemic," we cannot say for sure that voters are not also considering other factors that might influence their assessment of election integrity (i.e., some portion of voters who reported that they lack certainty about whether their vote will be counted accurately in light of the pandemic might have had similar concerns about election integrity even in the absence of a pandemic).

As discussed in the previous section, we considered the demographic, attitudinal, and geographic factors that are likeliest to predict whether respondents expected their vote to be counted accurately. We categorized voters into two groups: those who responded "yes" (we label these individuals as certain about the integrity of the election) and those who responded "no" or "unsure" (we label these individuals as uncertain). Again, we used statistical analysis to identify characteristics associated with perceptions of integrity.[9] The results of this analysis are presented in Box 2.2.

There is a strong relationship between perception of safety, discussed in the previous section, and perception of integrity regarding the November 2020 election. Those respondents who reported certainty that the election would be free of physical health risks related to the pandemic also reported certainty that their ballot would be counted accurately, even when taking into account demographic, partisan, and regional effects. Similarly, respondents who reported that local officials were more prepared to safeguard their health in the 2020 election (*perception of preparedness*) were more likely to also report believing that their votes would be counted accurately.

---

[9] We used a logistic regression. Details on the method are provided in the appendix.

BOX 2.2

Demographic and Geographic Factors Associated with Perception of Integrity

Characteristics associated with perception of integrity:

- age**
- Republican (compared with Democrat)**
- male (compared with female)***
- higher level of education (postgraduate degree compared with less than college)***
- expect election to be safe***
- voted in 2016 and/or 2018**
- believe local officials are prepared***
- live in the Midwest (compared with Northeast)**

Characteristics associated with uncertainty about integrity:

- Hispanic**
- Black/African American*** (compared with White/Caucasian)

* $p < 0.05$ (moderate statistical significance); ** $p < 0.01$ (high statistical significance); *** $p < 0.001$ (very high statistical significance).
NOTES: Survey question was phrased as "Do you feel that your vote will be counted accurately in light of the current pandemic?" These models are unweighted but results from weighted models were substantively the same. As a robustness check, we also ran models that exclude the other perception variables (e.g., looking at perception of safety without including perception of integrity or preparedness). We found the results mostly unchanged. For details, see the appendix.

Partisanship and vote history are also relevant to perception of integrity. First, we found that Republicans are less likely than Democrats to report that they expect their vote to be counted accurately. But we also found that this relationship seems considerably weaker than that observed for safety, suggesting that partisan differences on perception of integrity are considerably less than was the case for perception of safety. In other words, although there appears to be a sizable number of Republican voters who believe that elections will be physically safe but that their vote will not be counted accurately, there are also Republicans who follow the more general pattern already noted of expecting both safety and election integrity.[10] Second, we found that those who voted in 2016 or 2018 are more likely to expect that their vote will be counted accurately in 2020.

Several other demographic factors also appear to be associated with perceptions of integrity:

- Women appeared less likely than men to expect that their votes will be counted accurately within the pandemic context.
- Older respondents and those with higher levels of education appeared more likely than younger respondents and those with lower levels of education to expect that their votes will be counted accurately.
- We also found differences across race or ethnic group. Black respondents and Hispanic respondents were less likely than White respondents and non-Hispanic respondents to report that they expect that their ballots will be counted accurately.

We again used our analysis to consider how reported perception of safety varies across demographic characteristics identified in Box 2.2 (see Figure 2.2[11]). We conducted this analysis only for those

---

[10] This assessment is supported by robustness checks, which show that partisanship is no longer a statistically significant predictor of perceptions of integrity in some models. For details, see the appendix.

[11] As with Figure 2.1, Figure 2.2 reports predicted probabilities, which are the statistical model's predictions about how the average person who matches the group of interest would respond to the question about the integrity of the 2020 election (i.e., how likely the average

variables found to meaningfully influence reported perceptions of integrity. Results use population weights. A few relationships are worth highlighting:

- For respondents who reported voting in 2016 and/or 2018, we predict that 72 percent would report that they expect their vote to be counted accurately, compared with only 44 percent of those who did not vote in those years.
- The model indicates that among Black/African American respondents, 45 percent would report that they expect their vote to be counted accurately compared to 71 percent among White/Caucasian respondents.
- The relevance of perceptions of safety and preparedness to perceptions of integrity again stands out. The model predicts that, among those who reported confidence in the preparedness of local officials, 48 percent would also report confidence in election integrity, compared with 79 percent for those who lack certainty in election preparedness.

Assessments of Local Official Preparedness

Finally, we asked respondents, *"Do you believe your local elections officials are prepared to safeguard your physical health from risks associated with COVID-19 during the 2020 presidential election?"* (we call this *perception of preparedness*, as mentioned in the previous section). About 55 percent of respondents reported that they felt that local officials are prepared to protect voters from risks to their physical safety. About 17 percent felt that local officials are not prepared, and about 28 percent

person would be to respond yes or no/unsure). For example, the comparison between voters in 2016 and 2018 and those who did not vote in those years assesses the average respondent in each group; the assessment would therefore incorporate the fact that frequent voters tend to be older than infrequent voters and that minority groups tend to turn out at lower rates than nonminority voters. Predicted probabilities use population weights. All variables illustrated were shown to have independent effects above and beyond other characteristics (i.e., they are identified in the statistical model as being statistically significant).

Figure 2.2
Predicted Percentage of Agreement with Perception of Integrity Survey Question

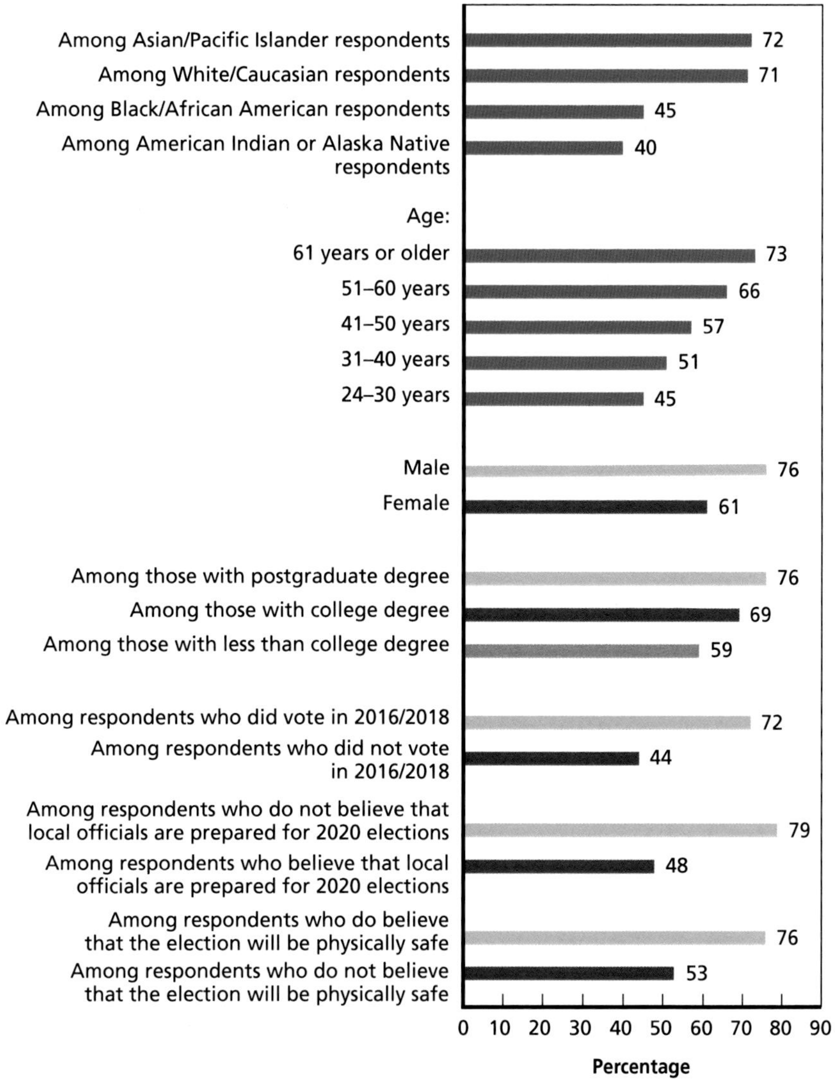

NOTE: Survey question phrasing was "Do you feel that your vote will be counted accurately in light of the current pandemic?" Predicted probabilities use population weights.

were not sure. In addition to descriptive analysis, we used a statistical model to identify demographic, geographic, and political preference characteristics associated with respondents' views of local preparedness.[12] We categorized voters into two groups: those who responded "yes" (we label these individuals as certain about the preparedness of local officials) and those who responded "no" or "unsure" (we label these individuals as uncertain about the preparedness of local officials). Again, we started by considering the geographic, demographic, and political preference characteristics that are associated with perception of the preparedness of local officials. Results appear in Box 2.3.

Once again, we found that partisanship and voting history were among the most significant and meaningful factors. Republicans, compared with Democrats and independents, were more likely to express confidence in officials' preparedness. There is also some evidence that those who reported voting absentee or by mail in the 2016 or 2018 elections might be somewhat less certain about the preparedness of local officials to safeguard their health than those who voted in person.

Considering demographic characteristics, we found that older respondents were more likely than younger ones to express that they believe that local officials are prepared. We also found that male respondents were less likely than female respondents to report that they believe that local officials are prepared, but we did not find differences by race or ethnicity. Neither are there significant differences stemming from respondents' regions of residence. We found that voters who live in urban areas were less likely than rural respondents to report that they think that local officials are prepared. We also note that respondents with higher levels of education appeared less likely to report that they expect local officials to be prepared to safeguard health than was the case for respondents with lower levels of education.

Finally, we found a correlation between perception of preparedness and other assessments of risk regarding personal health safety and election integrity. Respondents who expressed a lack of certainty about safety and integrity also expressed a lack of certainty about local official preparedness. This suggests that some individuals have

---

[12] Specifically, we used a logistic regression. Full results are included in the appendix.

BOX 2.3

Demographic and Geographic Factors Associated with Perception of Preparedness

Characteristics associated with perception of preparedness:

- age***
- Republican (compared with Democrat)*
- believe election will be safe***
- expect vote to be counted***

Characteristics associated with uncertainty about preparedness:

- male (compared with female)*
- higher level of education (postgraduate compared with less than college)*
- voted by mail or absentee in last election***
- live in urban region (compared with rural)**

* $p < 0.05$ (moderate statistical significance); ** $p < 0.01$ (high statistical significance); *** $p < 0.001$ (very high statistical significance).
NOTES: Survey question was phrased as "Do you believe your local elections officials are prepared to safeguard your physical health from risks associated with COVID-19 during the 2020 presidential election?" These models are unweighted but results from weighted models were substantively the same. As a robustness check, we also ran models that exclude the other perception variables (e.g., looking at perception of safety without including perception of integrity or preparedness). We found the results mostly unchanged. For details, see the appendix.

more-optimistic overall assessments about the safe and secure execution of the November 2020 election.

To further extend this analysis, we consider how beliefs about the preparedness of local officials to safeguard health in the November election vary across the groups identified as significant in Box 2.3

(see Figure 2.3[13]). Results use predicted percentages from the regression model. A few relationships are worth highlighting:

- For those who said they believed that the 2020 general election will be physically safe, the model predicts that 76 percent would also report that local officials will safeguard their health, compared with only 35 percent of those who did not express certainty about the safety of the election.
- The influence of partisanship is also clear, especially comparing those who identified themselves as Democrats with those who identified themselves as Republicans. Among Democrats, the model predicts that 60 percent would report believing that local officials are prepared to safeguard their health; while this prediction is 78 percent among Republicans.
- The model predicts that the belief that local officials are prepared will be most likely among those who previously voted in person compared with those who voted by mail.
- We also found differences across age groups: The model expects older respondents to be more likely to express confidence in the preparedness of local officials to safeguard health in November.

Preferred Mitigations

To further explore the concept of preparedness, we asked respondents what type of mitigations they felt election officials should take to safeguard the physical health of voters. We asked about three measures:

---

[13] Figure 2.3 reports predicted probabilities, which are the statistical model's predictions about how the average person who matches the group of interest would respond to the question about the preparedness of election officials for the 2020 election (i.e., how likely the average person would be to respond yes or no/unsure). For example, a comparison between voters in 2016 and 2018 and those who did not vote in those years assesses the average respondent in each group; the assessment would therefore incorporate the fact that frequent voters tend to be older than infrequent voters and that minority groups tend to turn out at lower rates than nonminority voters. All variables illustrated were shown to have independent effects above and beyond other characteristics (i.e., they are identified in the statistical model as being statistically significant).

Figure 2.3
Predicted Percentage of Agreement with Perception of Preparedness Survey Question

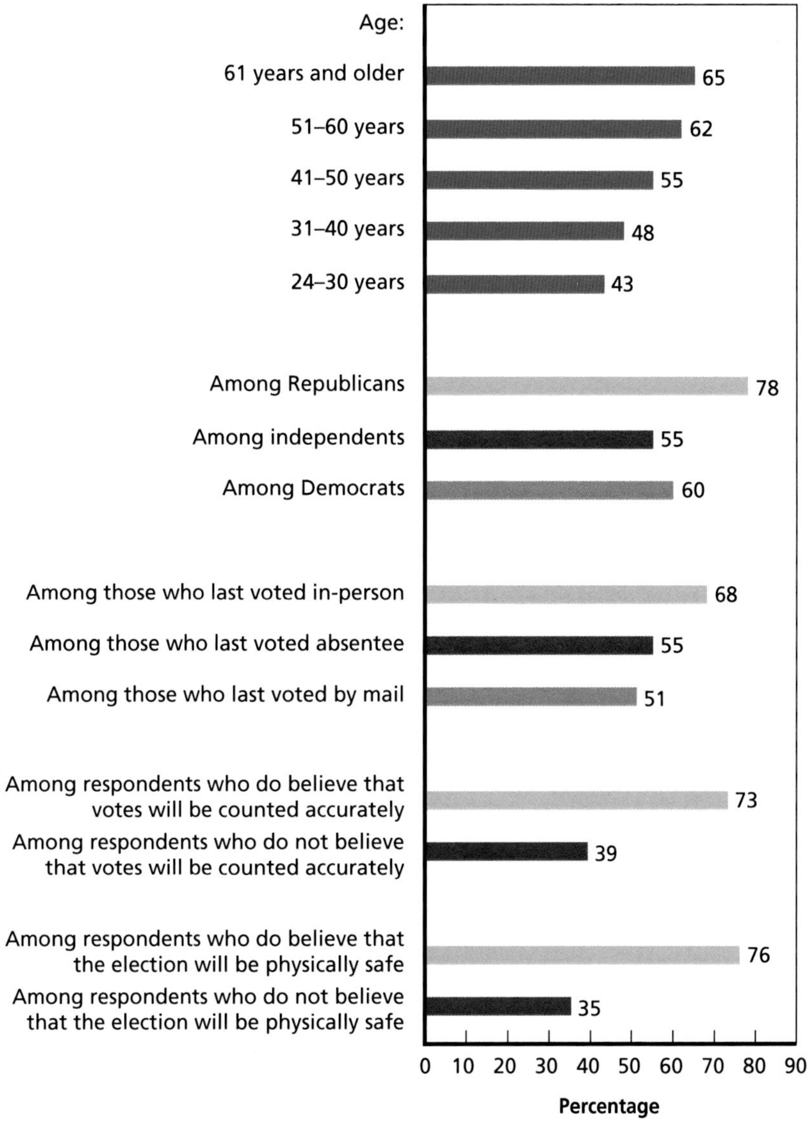

NOTES: Survey question was phrased as "Do you believe your local elections officials are prepared to safeguard your physical health from risks associated with COVID-19 during the 2020 presidential election?" Predicted probabilities use population weights.

social distancing and sanitization at the polls, distribution of mail-in ballots to all registered voters, and online voting. Respondents were able to express support for none, one, some, or all of the measures. To explore factors that influenced respondent choices on these measures, support for each measure was modeled independently using a statistical model that featured demographic, geographic, and political preference characteristics.[14]

There was wide agreement among respondents that, of the three options provided, states should use social distancing and sanitize polling places. Eighty-three percent of respondents reported that they supported the use of sanitation and social distancing, and only 17 percent expressed a lack of support for this measure. On the other hand, 53 percent said that all registered voters should be provided mail-in ballots, and only 34 percent felt that local election officials should pursue online voting.

Voters' assessments of the types of safeguards that local officials should take to ensure the physical safety of the November elections appeared to be shaped by many of the same factors that seemingly influenced their perceptions of safety and integrity. For example, support for different measures varied depending on partisanship. All things considered, Republicans were predicted to be uniquely more likely to support social distancing and sanitation at the polls than Democrats and independents and to be more opposed than Democrats or independents to expanded distribution of mail-in ballots to all registered voters and online voting.

In terms of geographic differences, urban voters were more likely than their rural counterparts to support expanded distribution of mail-in ballots to registered voters and online voting measures (net of partisan, demographic, and regional considerations). Respondents living in the West were more likely than those in the Northeast to express support for expanded distribution of mail-in ballots (given that several Western states already have universal mail-in options, this might be because of their experience with this voting method), but less likely

[14] Specifically, we used a logistic regression with success measured as support for the measure.

to support online voting or sanitation and social distancing as mitigations. Somewhat surprisingly, however, respondents who live in states that already offer a no-excuse mail-in option are less likely than others to support expanded distribution of mail-in ballots and online voting, perhaps because they already have easy access to mail-in ballots and see it as unnecessary.

Education seemed to have less effect on mitigation preferences, although respondents reporting having higher levels of education showed slightly more support for both social distancing and sanitation practices and expanded distribution of mail-in ballots to registered voters. Older voters were less likely to support social distancing and online voting (net of other partisan, regional, and demographic considerations); they did not differ from younger voters on average in supporting expanded access to mail-in ballots for registered voters.

Finally, we found few differences by race or ethnicity. Respondents who identified themselves as Hispanic appeared less likely to support expanded distribution of mail-in ballots (the same is true of Black/African American respondents compared with White respondents) but more supportive than non-Hispanic respondents of online voting.

These results are summarized in Table 2.2.

Summary

We can draw some comparisons across these three analyses about factors that appear relevant to perceptions of safety, election integrity, and preparedness. First, age appears to matter. Despite the higher risk that COVID-19 poses to older voters, this group generally has more-positive perceptions of safety, election integrity, and preparedness than do younger voters. This might reflect the fact that, in recent decades, older Americans have generally tended to have greater trust in government institutions than younger Americans.[15] We also found that there

[15] Russell J. Dalton, "The Social Transformation of Trust in Government," *International Review of Sociology*, Vol. 15, No. 1, 2005; Lee Rainie, Scott Keeter, and Andrew Perrin, "Trust and Distrust in America," Pew Research Center, July 22, 2019.

Table 2.2
Characteristics Associated with Mitigation Options

Sanitation and Social Distancing		Expanded Distribution of Mail-In Ballots to Registered Voters		Online Voting	
Associated with Increased Support	**Associated with Decreased Support**	**Associated with Increased Support**	**Associated with Decreased Support**	**Associated with Increased Support**	**Associated with Decreased Support**
Republican (compared with Democrat)		Higher education (compared with less than college)	Republican (compared with Democrat)		Republican (compared with Democrat)
Higher education (compared with less than college)		Lives in West (compared with Northeast)	Hispanic	Hispanic	Lives in West or Midwest (compared with Northeast)
		Lives in urban area (compared with rural)	No-excuse mail-in option in the state	Lives in urban area (compared with rural)	Male (compared with female)
			Black/African American (compared with White/ Caucasian)		

NOTES: Survey question was phrased as "What measures do you think elections officials should take to safeguard your physical health from risks associated with COVID-19 during the 2020 presidential election?" The appendix lists the full results. These models are unweighted but results from weighted models were substantively the same.

are clear differences across racial or ethnic groups. We found that Black respondents tended to be less likely than White respondents to expect their votes to be counted accurately. Hispanic respondents were also less likely than non-Hispanic respondents to expect their votes to be counted accurately and to expect local officials to be prepared to safeguard health. Education also matters; voters who have higher levels of education are less likely to expect that elections will be physically safe but more likely to expect that their votes will be counted accurately.

We also found consistent differences across political parties and voting histories. Respondents who identified themselves as Democrats were consistently less likely than those who identified themselves as Republicans to report that they expect the election to be safe and that they expect election officials to be prepared to safeguard public health, but they were also somewhat more likely to expect that their votes will be counted accurately despite the pandemic. As noted previously, these differences likely reflect systematic differences among members of each partisan group in such areas as trust in institutions and attitudes toward the risk posed by COVID-19 generally, but the differences also might be influenced by the political discourse of party elites on each side of the aisle. Finally, voting history appears to matter. Respondents who reported voting in 2016 and/or 2018 appear to have universally more-positive assessments about the likely safety and integrity of the November 2020 election than respondents who did not vote in either of these two years (and so might be lapsed or traditionally nonvoters).

We also considered respondent attitudes toward mitigations and found that many of the same factors that seem to influence perceptions also appear to affect attitudes toward various mitigations. We note that self-identified Republicans are more likely to support sanitation and social distancing at the polls but less likely to support expanded distribution of mail-in ballots to all registered voters or online voting. Education also matters consistently; respondents with higher levels of education are more likely than those with lower levels of education to support both social distancing and sanitation practices at the polls and expanded distribution of mail-in ballots to all registered voters. Respondents who live in urban areas express higher support than rural respondents for both distribution of mail-in ballots to all registered voters and online voting. Finally, Hispanic and Black respondents are less supportive than non-Hispanic respondents and White respondents, respectively, of sending mail-in ballots to all registered voters; Hispanic respondents are, however, more supportive than non-Hispanic respondents of online voting.

Understanding the factors that shape perceptions of safety, election integrity, and preparedness can help election officials understand how to best allay public concerns and target messaging to ensure that voters feel safe and secure regardless of the trajectory of the pandemic. However, it is useful to look more carefully at how these perceptions influence intention to vote. It is possible that their influence is significant, in which case mitigation might be important. However, it is also possible that the relationship between perception and intention is marginal or is mediated by other factors. We turn to these questions in the next chapter.

CHAPTER THREE

How Do Perceptions Shape Intention to Vote?

In this chapter, we consider how perceptions of safety, election integrity, and preparedness influence intention to vote. In other words, are respondents who are more or less fearful about their physical safety or more or less concerned about election integrity more or less likely to vote as a result? To conduct this analysis, we reviewed what past research says about these questions and then applied the key hypotheses emerging from this literature to our own data. We also look at *how* people plan to vote and whether the pandemic seems to be driving a shift away from in-person voting.

What We Know from Past Research

There is a large body of literature that considers the factors that shape an individual's *intention to vote*, or their own assessment of their likelihood of going to the polls to participate in an election. Research on intention to vote underscores several key insights. First, voters who assess their intention to be high are the most likely to actually turn out, but there is also significant attrition between intention and reality. In other words, some percentage of people who say they are nearly certain to vote in a coming election ultimately might not turn out to vote when that election occurs.[1] Second, the literature high-

[1] Christopher H. Achen and André Blais, "Intention to Vote, Reported Vote, and Validated Vote," in Johan A. Elkink and David M. Farrell, eds., *The Act of Voting: Identities, Institutions and Locale*, London: Routledge, 2015; William A. Glaser, "Intention and Voting Turnout,"

lights some of the demographic factors most likely to shape intention to vote. Men, older voters, voters with higher education levels and incomes, self-identified Republicans, and White voters are more likely to report high intention to vote and more likely to actually vote than the corresponding comparison groups (women, younger voters, those with lower education levels and incomes, self-identified Democrats, and minorities).[2] In our analysis, we compare our results with these findings to assess our consistency with past research.

There has been less research into factors that shape how voters intend to cast ballots. We can, however, draw on past analysis that considers which types of voters are most likely to vote by mail to get some sense of whether we should expect specific types of voters to be more or less likely to vote by mail or to shift to voting by mail in the current context. First, most research indicates that mail-in voting is more effective at retaining past voters than it is at mobilizing new voters.[3] Those most likely to take advantage of mail-in voting options tend to be people who were likely to vote anyway—the convenience of mail-in voting further bolsters the likelihood that they will vote. The addition of mail-in voting options does not, however, appear to expand the electorate by attracting previous nonvoters. For the most part, mail-in voters are not demographically different from voters who vote on Election Day; rather, they are a cross-section of the larger pool of voters.[4] Other studies indicate that those most likely to vote by mail tend to be older and White, to have higher education levels, and to be employed.[5] Second, existing research generally reports no partisan

---

American Political Science Review, Vol. 52, No. 4, 1958; Donald Granberg and Soren Holmberg, "Self-Reported Turnout and Voter Validation," *American Journal of Political Science*, Vol. 35, No. 2, 1991.

2 Achen and Blais, 2015; Glaser, 1958; Granberg and Holmberg, 1991.

3 Adam J. Berinsky, Nancy Burns, and Michael W. Traugott, "Who Votes by Mail? A Dynamic Model of the Individual-Level Consequences of Voting-by-Mail Systems," *Public Opinion Quarterly*, Vol. 65, No. 2, 2001.

4 Priscilla L. Southwell and Justin I. Burchett, "The Effect of All-Mail Elections on Voter Turnout," *American Politics Quarterly*, Vol. 28, No. 1, 2000.

5 Jeffrey A. Dubin and Gretchen A. Kalsow, "Comparing Absentee and Precinct Voters: A View over Time," *Political Behavior*, Vol. 18, No. 4, 1996.

effects—Republicans and Democrats are equally likely to choose vote-by-mail options.[6] Notably, this finding (that members of each party use vote-by-mail options at about the same rate) has continued to hold up through recent elections, even as the issue of mail-in voting has become increasingly politicized.[7]

Our analysis is specifically focused on how perceptions of safety, election integrity, and preparedness in the pandemic context might shape intention to vote above and beyond the demographic characteristics considered in most research. Some past research considers how threats to physical safety and assessments of integrity might affect turnout; the majority of work in this area focuses on non-U.S. contexts. Most existing analysis that considers physical safety discusses election violence and its effect on turnout. Most studies, including one focused on the effect of lynchings on the participation of Black voters in the post-Reconstruction U.S. South, have found that pre-election violence deters voters and reduces voter turnout, particularly among those groups targeted by the violence.[8] The threat of COVID-19 is more diffuse than the threat of election violence, but we would expect, based on past research, that those who perceive a physical health threat from the pandemic will have lower intention to vote, all else being equal. On the issue of election integrity, the effects are more mixed. In general, turnout is higher for elections that are perceived to have high integrity, meaning that voters have high confidence that the process

---

[6] Berinsky, Burns, and Traugott, 2001.

[7] For example, see Kevin Morris, "Who Votes by Mail?" Brennan Center for Justice, April 15, 2020; Daniel M. Thompson, Jennifer Wu, Jesse Yoder, and Andrew B. Hall, *The Neutral Partisan Effects of Vote-by-Mail: Evidence from County-Level Roll-Outs*, Palo Alto, Calif.: Stanford Institute for Economic Policy Research, Working Paper 20-015, 2020a; Daniel M. Thompson, Jennifer Wu, Jesse Yoder, and Andrew B. Hall, "Universal Vote-by-Mail Has No Impact on Partisan Turnout or Vote Share," *Proceedings of the National Academy of Sciences*, Vol. 117, No. 25, 2020b.

[8] Paul Collier and Pedro C. Vicente, "Votes and Violence: Evidence from a Field Experiment in Nigeria," *Economic Journal*, Vol. 124, No. 574, 2014; Daniel B. Jones, Werner Troesken, and Randall Walsh, "Political Participation in a Violent Society: The Impact of Lynching on Voter Turnout in the Post-Reconstruction South," *Journal of Development Economics*, Vol. 129, 2017; Alejandro Trelles and Miguel Carreras, "Bullets and Votes: Violence and Electoral Participation in Mexico," *Journal of Politics in Latin America*, Vol. 4, No. 2, 2012.

will be fair and transparent and that their votes will be counted accurately.[9] However, there are also cases in which overt threats to integrity, such as voter harassment, might actually motivate higher turnout.[10] The type and severity of threats and the extent to which voters feel that these threats to legitimacy can be overcome likely affect outcomes. Our expectation is that the effect of pandemic-related concern over election integrity on voter turnout will be rather weak. Generally speaking, we expect that those who have confidence in the integrity of the election despite the pandemic will be most likely to turn out.

In the following section, we consider intention to vote in the November 2020 election among respondents, focusing on how demographic and geographic characteristics and perceptions of safety and integrity are associated with intention to vote. We then make some historical comparisons regarding how intention to vote might have changed since 2016 for 2020 survey respondents and how expected methods of voting differ from those that respondents reported using in past elections.

Intention to Vote in November 2020

We asked respondents to report their intention to vote in November 2020 on a scale of 0 to 100, with 100 being certain to vote and 0 indicating that the respondent is certain not to vote. In response, a large number of respondents expressed that they were nearly certain to vote. As noted, people might overestimate the likelihood that they will vote.[11]

---

[9] Sarah Birch, "Perceptions of Electoral Fairness and Voter Turnout," *Comparative Political Studies*, Vol. 43, No. 12, 2010; Miguel Carreras and Yasemin İrepoğlu, "Trust in Elections, Vote Buying, and Turnout in Latin America," *Electoral Studies*, Vol. 32, No. 4, 2013; Ferran Martinez i Coma and Minh Trinh, "How Electoral Integrity Affects Voter Turnout in Democracies," *Australian Journal of Political Science*, Vol. 52, No. 1, 2017.

[10] Martinez i Coma and Trinh, 2017.

[11] Intention to vote, measured here as a probabilistic behavioral expectation, can be considered closer to an actual behavior than a more traditional intention-to-vote question (e.g., a question that asks respondents to place their likelihood of voting on a Likert scale of unlikely to likely) because it allows the respondent to incorporate any expected barriers into their answer. Thus, they can report their *likelihood* of voting (accounting for barriers) and not just their intention (putting these barriers to the side). This is consistent with the Theory of

Furthermore, with the election still six months away at the time of this survey, an individual's intention to vote could change significantly in the intervening period. In our sample, 49 percent reported that their intention to vote was 100 percent, while another 16 percent reported likelihoods of 90 percent or higher. About 6 percent reported a likelihood of 0, and another 6 percent reported likelihoods of between 1 and 10 percent. This distribution (which uses population weights) is illustrated in Figure 3.1.

Next, we considered characteristics that appear to be associated with intention to vote. Our models were built by drawing on past research identifying those factors most strongly associated with intention to vote, but we also included several other variables. Most central to this analysis, we used the three perception variables drawn from our

Figure 3.1
November 2020 Intention to Vote

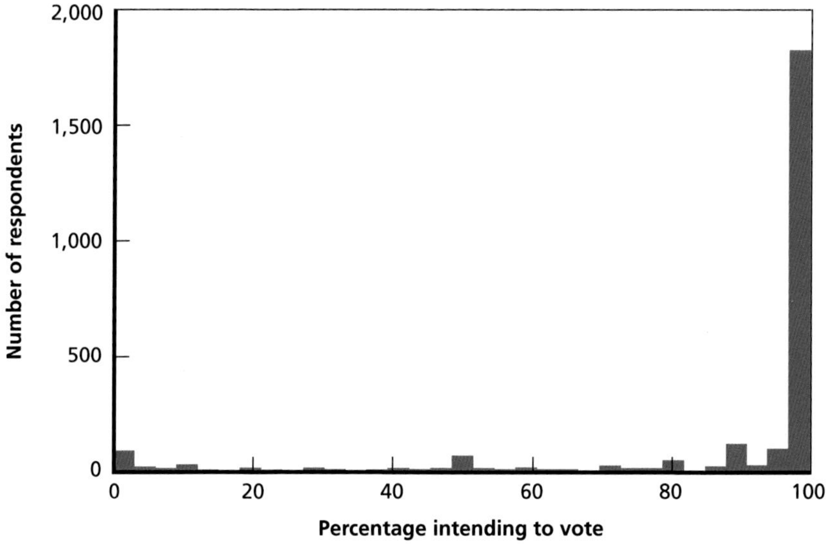

NOTE: Results use population weights.

Planned Behavior (for example, see Icek Ajzen, "From Intentions to Actions: A Theory of Planned Behavior," in Julius Kuhl and Jürgen Beckmann, eds., *Action Control: From Cognition to Behavior*, Berlin: Springer, 1985).

survey: perceptions of safety, integrity, and preparedness,[12] as well as geographic controls for region of the country and an indicator for states that have easy access to no-excuse mail-in voting (because these individuals might have different attitudes than those who have fewer remote-voting options). We used statistical analysis to explore characteristics associated with intention to vote. The dependent variable in this case broke respondents into three categories: certain or near certain not to vote (< 35 percent), uncertain whether they would vote (35–75 percent), and certain or near certain to vote (> 75 percent) in 2020.[13]

First, we considered individual and geographic characteristics and compared these with the findings of past research. Our results were broadly consistent with past research on intention to vote. All results are summarized in Box 3.1. We found the following:

- Reported intention to vote was highest for those with higher levels of education and lowest for those who had less than a college education.
- We found that Hispanic respondents reported lower intention to vote than non-Hispanic respondents, but we did not find differences by race.
- We found that respondents who reported having voted in 2016 and/or 2018 were likely to have higher intention to vote in the 2020 election than those who did not report voting in either year. This is consistent with literature showing that one of the strongest predictors of whether someone will vote is whether they have voted in the past.
- Respondents in urban areas expressed lower intention to vote than respondents in rural areas.
- We found little difference between Republicans and Democrats in terms of intention to vote, but found that independents reported lower intention to vote than either Democrats or Republicans.

---

[12] Although these three variables are closely related, we did not find significant concerns when featuring all three in one model. We explored models with only one perception variable at a time in the appendix.

[13] Full details on this model and others in this chapter are provided in the appendix.

BOX 3.1

Demographic, Attitudinal, and Geographic Factors Associated with Intention to Vote

Characteristics associated with higher intention to vote:

- voted in 2016 or 2018***
- believe election will be safe*
- higher level of education (compared with less than college)*

Characteristics associated with lower intention to vote:

- political affiliation reported as other or unsure***
- live in urban area (compared with rural)*
- Hispanic*

* $p < 0.05$ (moderate statistical significance); ** $p < 0.01$ (high statistical significance); *** $p < 0.001$ (very high statistical significance).
NOTES: Survey question was phrased as *"What is the percent chance that you will vote in the 2020 presidential election?"* Results do not use population weights but the weighted results are substantively the same. We found the results mostly unchanged. For details, see the appendix.

We also looked at our three variables of interest, those related to perceptions.[14] We found that perception of safety has a positive relationship with intention to vote: Those respondents who have confidence that voting in the election will not pose a risk to their physical health because of COVID-19 have higher intention to vote than those who expressed concerns about safety. Note that we make no causal claims; we can only suggest that perceptions of safety appear to be associated with intention to vote in a meaningful way. We did not find evidence that perceptions of preparedness have an independent positive

[14] We considered three different specifications: first, a model with all predictors and all three perception variables but no interactions; second, the same model with interactions to investigate conditional relationships; and third, three separate models, each with only one of the three perception variables. The results were largely consistent across models.

or negative effect on intention to vote over the full sample. Perceptions of integrity, in contrast, do not appear to be associated with intention to vote across the full the sample but might be relevant for certain subgroups, as we will describe. These results appear in Box 3.1.

Conditional Effects of Respondent Perceptions

The previous section explored average relationships of our three perception variables and vote intention, but we are also interested in whether perceptions of safety, election integrity, and preparedness have differential effects on different groups of voters. The perceived effects of these perceptions on intention to vote could differ by demographic group. For example, older populations might be more sensitive to perception of safety than younger ones because of their increased risk of death if they were to contract the disease. We used interaction effects to explore whether certain groups appear more or less sensitive to their perceptions of safety, election integrity, and preparedness.

Perception of Safety

As noted, our model predicts that voters who reported believing that their physical health will not be threatened by voting in November 2020 express higher intention to vote than those who report the opposite (that they fear COVID-19–related health threats as a consequence of voting). However, our analysis suggests that this effect differs depending on an individual's characteristics.

The most relevant demographic characteristics were race and ethnicity. For example, we found that, among respondents who do not feel that voting is safe, Black respondents were more likely to express higher intention to vote. Put another way, these individuals are less sensitive to their own perception of safety than comparison groups when expressing intention to vote. Alternatively, among respondents who reported confidence in the safety of voting, White respondents were more likely to report a high intention to vote (i.e., they appear more sensitive to perception of safety). This likely reflects the fact that a majority of voters do expect elections to be safe, combined with the facts that White respondents are more likely to fall into this group and that eligible voters who are White are significantly more likely to vote than minorities.

We found that other demographics did not seem to moderate this relationship between perception of safety and intention to vote. For instance, despite their higher risk of complications from the disease, perception of safety and intention to vote were not more closely related for older voters than for younger ones. Although this might be surprising based on what is known about elevated COVID-19–related risks among older populations, this finding might reflect the fact that older voters generally tend to show a higher commitment to voting than younger voters do.

Perception of Integrity

Although perception of integrity (whether respondents think their vote will be counted accurately) did not matter across all respondents, we found that respondents' perceptions about whether the pandemic would interfere with the counting of their ballot did influence intention to vote in certain cases. Among respondents who questioned the integrity of the 2020 election because of the pandemic, respondents with higher levels of education appear less likely to express high intention to vote; i.e., voters with lower levels of education who perceive election integrity to be high appear to be more likely to have high intention to vote, but those with higher levels of education are less sensitive to perception of integrity and, based on their assessment of integrity, might not adjust their expectations upward.

It is significant that the link between perception of integrity and intention to vote is conditional on education: That significance lies in what it suggests about how voting behavior might change among voters with lower levels of education who lose confidence in election integrity. Specifically, in a case where election integrity is questioned, our analysis indicates that voters with higher levels of education are likely to have little change in intention to vote, but those with lower levels of education would adjust their intention to vote. As election officials work to communicate that they are taking steps to reduce the public health risk, therefore, they might also need to communicate the steps they are taking to protect election integrity, such as setting up the infrastructure required to accurately count ballots of those who vote in person and by mail, and making particularly sure that this message reaches those voters with lower levels of education.

Perception of Preparedness

We did not find that perception of preparedness had significant conditional effects overall or for any subgroup, suggesting that assessment of local official preparedness does not seem to be related to intention to vote. Because perceptions of safety and integrity might be the factors with the most-direct implications for U.S. voters, they might have a closer tie to intention to vote than is the case for perception of preparedness.

Voting Intentions: Historical Comparisons

Although our analysis can tell us about factors likely to shape voting decisions in 2020, we can also use direct comparisons with respondent behavior in past elections to explore possible effects of the pandemic. Our analysis suggests that intention to vote might be reduced for those voters who have concerns about their physical safety at the polls and for some who are worried about the integrity of the election because of pandemic-related demands. In each case, the proportion of voters expressing concern about safety, election integrity, and preparedness is small, but the question remains: Should we be concerned that pandemic-related perceptions will significantly depress turnout? Although we cannot answer this question definitively, we can compare the intention to vote of respondents in our sample in May–June 2020 with these same individuals at a similar point in time: July–August 2016.[15] If we observe consistent declines in intention to vote between 2016 and 2020, then we might consider the pandemic as one possible driver of such a trend. We cannot prove such a hypothesis with the data at hand, nor can we predict whether behavior might change significantly closer to Election Day if pandemic conditions persist or worsen. But we can consider whether existing data are consistent with this explanation. On the other hand, if we see no major change or only minor changes, then

[15] As a reminder, intention to vote is a useful but not perfect predictor of actual turnout. Some potential voters might change their minds about voting as the election approaches; others might plan to vote but encounter some obstacle that prevents voting. Also relevant is that people tend to overestimate their likelihood of voting and to report that they voted even when they did not (see Achen and Blais, 2015).

we can take this as some evidence that the pandemic might not affect turnout. Of course, it is also possible that the pandemic itself has a depressing effect on intention to vote but that this effect is counterbalanced by other factors that increase intention to vote, such as enthusiasm about a specific candidate or issue.

Using a July–August 2016 survey conducted as part of the Presidential Election Panel Survey, we compared the May–June 2020 intention to vote data collected in our survey with those collected for the same respondents in July–August 2016.[16] We compared intention to vote across 2016 and 2020 in two ways. First, we assessed whether the distributions are the same or different considering only those respondents that appear in both data sets. We found that the distributions are different, but that intention to vote in 2020 appears slightly higher than intention to vote for the same respondents in 2016.[17]

Second, we looked at the proportion of voters who shift from being "certain or nearly certain to vote" to "uncertain" or "certain not to vote" and vice versa. We used the same definitions as previously, so respondents with an intention to vote that was higher than 75 percent were placed in the "certain or nearly certain to vote" group and the rest were grouped in the "not certain to vote" category. This plot is shown in Figure 3.2: Those who are certain or nearly certain to vote are shown on the top in green; those not certain to vote are on the bottom in red, where the size of each band indicates the number of voters. The curved bands highlight those respondents who switched categories. We can observe from this figure that only a small percentage of voters shifted from certain to uncertain; if anything, there is a stronger trend in the other direction of voters who appear more certain to vote in 2020 than they were at a similar time in 2016. There is little evidence, then, that the pandemic is leading to a decline in intention to vote, at least at the

---

[16] Pollard and Mendelsohn, 2016.

[17] We used a paired *t*-test, a statistical method for comparing observations on the same group made at separate times to see whether differences are statistically meaningful. This comparison considers only matched pairs, but an unpaired *t*-test to examine whether the 2016 and 2020 samples have different means similarly finds a statistically significant difference. The weighted mean for 2020 was 77.3 percent; that for 2016 was 70.3 percent.

Figure 3.2
Difference in Intention to Vote Between 2016 and 2020

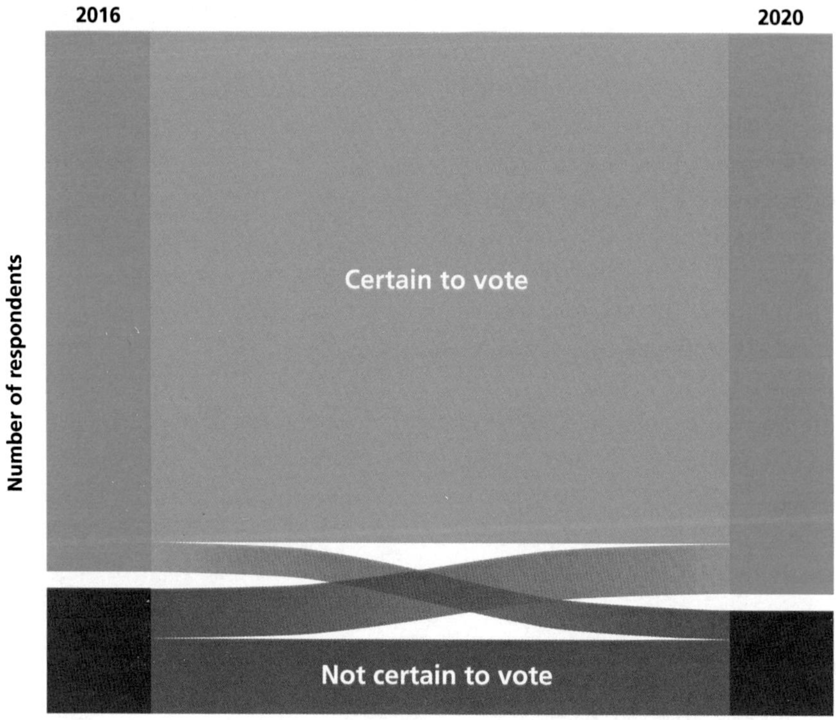

aggregate level.[18] Recent primary elections support this observation: Turnout in such states as Georgia and Kentucky has been higher in 2020 than in 2016, despite the pandemic context.[19]

We also considered changes in intention to vote by looking at which groups are more or less likely to shift from "certain to vote" in the 2016 survey to "uncertain to vote" or "certain not to vote" in 2020. Although individuals might make this choice for any number of reasons, one pos-

---

[18] We can also look at the aggregate proportion of voters that appear in the "certain to vote" category. Using population weights, we found that 68.4 percent of respondents in 2020 fall in this category, compared with 65 percent in 2016.

[19] Dareh Gregorian, "Voter Turnout Soared in Georgia, Despite Massive Primary Day Problems," NBC News, June 12, 2020; Sarah Ewall Wice, "Kentucky on Track for Historic Turnout," CBS News, June 23, 2020.

sibility is concern about election safety or preparedness. We used statistical analysis using interaction effects between intention to vote in 2016 and demographic, geographic, and partisan characteristics to estimate separately how well past intention to vote predicts future intention to vote within each subgroup. Full results are shown in the appendix. Among those who reported that they were certain to vote in 2016, our model predicted the following:

- no differences along partisanship, region of residence, or race or ethnicity among those whose intention to vote declined and those for whom it did not, although respondents who did not identify a party affiliation do seem significantly less likely to report high intention to vote in 2020
- respondents who reported believing that local officials are prepared to safeguard health are likely to report continued high intention to vote in 2020
- respondents with higher levels of education are more likely to report continued high intention to vote in 2020 than those with lower levels of education
- older respondents are less likely than younger ones to report the same high intention to vote between 2016 and 2020. (This might relate to the health-risk correlation with age and likelihood of voting that we noted previously. This result could suggest that although there is no such relationship across all voters, some older voters might have weakened in their intention to vote as a result of the pandemic.)

Vote Method

One explanation for the limited change in overall intention to vote between 2016 and 2020 might be that voters have changed how they plan to vote but not whether they plan to vote. To assess this hypothesis, we compared how respondents said they plan to vote in 2020 with how they reported voting in their most recent previous election. Here, we did find some notable differences. At an aggregate level, a smaller percentage of respondents reported that they are likely to vote in person than reported having done so in their last election—55 percent versus

69 percent—and 45 percent plan to vote remotely (compared with 31 percent in the last election). Although this shift could be because of changing norms or even changing policies, it is also possible that the shift is partly attributable to the pandemic context. It is notable that the percentage of voters who have voted by mail has increased steadily in presidential elections over the past three decades (from 7.8 percent in 1996 to almost 21 percent in 2016).[20] A more detailed look at this apparent shift reveals 389 voters who switched from voting in person to a vote-by-mail option or vice versa. Of this, 310 voters switched from "vote in person," to a remote, vote-by-mail option (about 12 percent of the total sample, but almost 80 percent of the switchers), while 79 (about 20 percent of the switchers) shifted from a remote voting option to voting in person. Again, this shift could be driven by any number of concurrent factors but might be at least partly driven by concerns about the pandemic and its implications for in-person voting. Figure 3.3 shows this shift of a sizable portion of voters from voting in person to intention to vote by mail in 2020.

Finally, we wanted to observe the demographic, geographic, and attitudinal characteristics of respondents who reported that they intend to vote by mail in 2020 but reported voting in person in their last election. In other words, we wanted to know whether certain types of people were most likely to make this shift. We used statistical analysis to explore the characteristics of those most likely to indicate that they planned to switch from voting in person to a vote-by-mail option in 2020.[21] Our findings were as follows:

- Again, partisanship is a substantial predictor; our model indicates that Republican respondents are much less likely than Democratic ones to make the switch from in-person voting to mail-in voting.
- Those respondents who reported that they expect voting will be safe are much less likely to switch from in-person to mail-in voting, which is consistent with what we would expect if pandemic-related

---

[20] Hannah Hartig, Bradley Jones, and Vianney Gomez, "As States Move to Expand the Practice, Relatively Few Americans Have Voted by Mail," Pew Research Center, June 24, 2020.

[21] We again used logistic regression. Full results are in the appendix.

Figure 3.3
Difference in Intended Voting Method in 2020

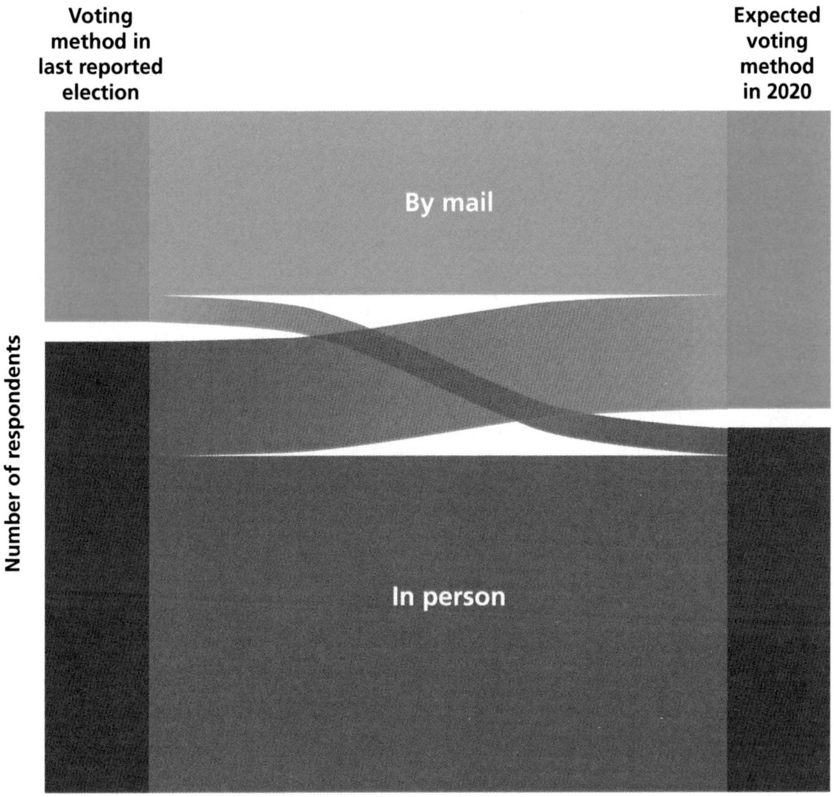

concern is a factor driving respondent choices in this case. Similarly, our model predicts that those who reported holding the opposite perception about safety are more likely to shift to remote voting options. This is a significant finding; it suggests that eligible voters do see remote voting options as a way to mitigate safety risk from the pandemic.

- Those who reside in the West were uniquely more likely to switch to vote-by-mail options than those in other regions, perhaps because of easier access to such options in that region.
- Interestingly, those who reside in states without a no-excuse mail-in option were more likely to report intention to switch; absent

an unobserved reason why respondents might report a genuine excuse to vote by mail, these respondents might be surprised to find restrictions in place that prevent them from receiving a mail-in ballot. There are a significant number of these individuals in the data: About 80 percent of those who intend to switch from in-person voting to a vote-by-mail option live in a state where an excuse is required to vote by mail. It is possible that these voters anticipate a temporary policy change that allows them to vote remotely in 2020 because of COVID-19 concerns.

- Respondents who did not vote in 2016 and/or 2018 and those who live in urban areas (compared with rural areas) are more likely to intend to switch to a vote-by-mail option.
- Interestingly, age has no significant effect beyond the characteristics observed here, despite higher health risks for older voters.

Summary

Our analyses suggest that perception of safety appears to be associated with intention to vote for the average voter (i.e., those who feel safer are more likely to vote), although it seems to matter somewhat less for Black respondents than for White respondents. Perception of integrity matters for select groups of voters, especially those with higher levels of education. We found little evidence at the aggregate level that the pandemic is having a strong depressing effect on anticipated turnout. We also illustrate a notable shift among voters who previously voted in person who expressed an intention to vote by mail, perhaps as a response to the pandemic: Those respondents who perceived the election to be less safe were more likely to switch from in-person to mail-in voting.

Of all perception-related variables, we found that perception of safety is most important to intention to vote, although we observed previously that perception of safety is closely associated with perceptions of integrity and preparedness. Election officials might need to focus specific attention on safety but should also consider ways to communicate their preparedness to conduct the election in a way that protects security and privacy.

CHAPTER FOUR

Conclusions and Implications

In this report, we have considered attitudes about the safety and integrity of elections in November 2020 and the preparedness of local officials to manage elections in the pandemic context. We also explored how these perceptions are related to intention to vote.

The most notable observation is that the majority of respondents said that they expect that the 2020 election will be physically safe from COVID-19 health risks, that their votes will be counted accurately despite the challenges of the pandemic, and that local officials are prepared to carry out elections successfully despite the additional challenges. Equally important, however, is that, in each case, about one-third of respondents reported that they are "unsure" about safety, election integrity, or preparedness. Combined with the smaller percentages who feel certain that the election will not be physically safe in terms of their health, that their vote will not be counted accurately, or that local officials will not be prepared to safeguard their health, this amounts to a sizable portion of potential voters who have pandemic-related concerns about the November 2020 election. Furthermore, we found a clear relationship among the three perceptions. This means that for voters who do not expect elections to be safe, their vote to be counted accurately, or election officials to be prepared, these concerns extend across dimensions. Election officials and other stakeholders involved in election administration might be able to counter this uncertainty through strategic and extensive communication about the steps they are taking to prepare and to ensure sufficient sanitation, the needed number of pollworkers, and the necessary technology to manage secure elections with a sizable remote component. Health and integrity concerns need to be addressed simultaneously.

Our analyses also highlighted some relevant cross-group differences in perceptions that might be relevant to the crafting and dissemination of such strategic messages. First, we found significant partisan differences. Self-identified Republicans were more likely to express expectations of safety and preparedness but also somewhat more likely to express concern about integrity than was the case for self-identified Democrats. We also found that older voters, all else being equal, expressed higher expectations of safety and preparedness and were more likely to say that they believed their votes would be counted accurately than was the case for younger voters. Race and ethnicity were also significant and relevant. We found that Black respondents tended to express less confidence in election integrity and in the preparedness of local officials than was the case for White respondents. Hispanic respondents were also less likely than non-Hispanic respondents to say that they expected local officials to be adequately prepared.

We found that voters also differed in their assessments of various mitigations: Sanitation and social distancing at the polls received the most support, followed by the widespread dissemination of mail-in ballots to all registered voters and online voting. Although support for social distancing and sanitation was broad, respondents with higher levels of education and those who lived in urban areas were more likely than respondents with lower income levels or those who lived in rural areas to support expanded distribution of mail-in ballots to all registered voters. Support for online voting was low, especially among male respondents and Republican respondents.

These results are not generally surprising, given what we know about the attitudes of different groups toward COVID-19 and their trust in institutions. For example, we have noted that past surveys demonstrate the greater concern about COVID-19 among Democrats and the greater trust in institutions among older voters that might bolster their trust in the preparedness of local officials. Similarly, we know from past research that racial and ethnic minorities tend to have less trust in institutions because of a history of discrimination.[1] The most unexpected finding was that respondents who reported voting by mail in their last election were the least likely to expect that local officials would be prepared to safeguard health in 2020. This might be the result of some unobserved characteristic of individuals who are more prone to these types of concerns that also makes them more likely to vote by mail. It might be worth continuing to track these voters to see whether this relationship holds in the future.

We then considered how perceptions of safety, election integrity, and preparedness are associated with intention to vote. In the aggregate, we found little evidence that intention to vote is significantly lower among our group of respondents than was the case at a similar point in 2016. We found only a small number of respondents who responded to both a 2016 survey and our 2020 survey who reported large changes in their intention to vote. However, we did find a notable increase in the number of respondents planning to vote by mail rather than in person as they reported doing in their most recent past election. Rather than deciding not to vote, then, many respondents seem to be making plans to vote using remote methods.

Although perception of safety has a positive relationship with intention to vote, we found little independent relationship between intention to vote and perceptions of election integrity and preparedness. However, perceptions of safety, election integrity, and preparedness were all clearly related to each other: For example, individuals for whom safety concerns reduce their intention to vote might also have concerns about integrity and preparedness that further depress their intention to vote. We also observed that safety and integrity matter more to intention to vote for some voters than others. For example, Black respondents seem less influenced by their perception of safety than White respondents. Respondents with higher levels of education appear similarly less strongly influenced by their assessments of election integrity. These differential effects underscore that not everyone responds in the same ways to concerns about pandemic-related safety, election integrity, and preparedness. These differences might reflect

---

1 Jeffrey W. Koch, "Racial Minorities' Trust in Government and Government Decision-makers," *Social Science Quarterly*, Vol. 100, No. 1, 2019.

individual commitment to voting as a civic duty or a motivation to vote in 2020 driven by specific candidates or issues.

This survey reflects respondent attitudes a full five months before the election, providing a baseline, not an endpoint, for understanding the relationship between perceptions of safety, election integrity, and preparedness and intention to vote. Not only will respondent attitudes and perceptions likely change, but the trajectory of the virus itself is similarly uncertain. Perceptions of safety, for example, can change significantly, and respondents' attitudes at the time of the survey might reflect assumptions about the pandemic abating that might not hold true if the pandemic continues or intensifies in the fall. Continuing to track perceptions of safety, election integrity, and preparedness and how they are associated with intention to vote will be useful for election officials and other stakeholders seeking to determine whether their efforts to reassure voters and to prevent pandemic-related declines in turnout are having the desired effects.

Implications

The analyses in this report yield several useful observations for policymakers and election officials as they plan for the November 2020 election.

Intention to Vote Seems Robust to Pandemic Concerns

Although there is some evidence that safety concerns are associated with lower intention to vote, there is little evidence that voters are significantly less likely to vote in this pandemic context than they were in 2016. At least some portion of the stability in voter intention to vote might reflect respondents' expectations about steps that local officials will take to mitigate risk. Failure to then take those steps and to communicate with the public about ongoing preparations could result in a different outcome than expected.

Ensuring and Messaging a Commitment to Both Safety and Integrity Will Be Important

Our analyses indicate that perception of safety is more strongly related to intention to vote, but that perception of integrity also matters to some groups. Election integrity is a key concern in all elections and can encompass everything from protecting against cyber threats and voter fraud to ensuring voter privacy, but the pandemic context will bring additional logistical challenges, especially in places where the volume of mail-in ballots is expected to be significantly greater than usual (straining available resources) or where staffing sufficient polling places will make in-person voting more difficult. Election officials who are interested in ensuring that those who would otherwise vote are not deterred from doing so in 2020 because of pandemic-related concerns should ensure that they prioritize safety and election integrity equally and that they clearly communicate with constituents about the steps being taken. This could mean additional investments in equipment or larger efforts to recruit additional pollworkers or acquire protective gear for pollworkers.

Offering No-Excuse Mail-In Options Could Mitigate Safety Concerns

We found that voters who live in Western states that offer no-excuse mail-in options were more likely to report that they expected the 2020 general election to be free from health-related risks. We also observed that respondents who did not report an expectation that the 2020 election would be free from health concerns were more likely to report an intention to switch to mail-in voting. We cannot make causal arguments, but this result at least suggests that states interested in mitigating the safety concerns of voters should consider offering a no-excuse mail-in option if one does not already exist. It is worth noting that only 16 states do not have such an option—and several of these (for example, Massachusetts, Arkansas, and Connecticut) implemented a no-excuse provision for 2020.[2] Choosing to shift to a no-excuse mail-in system does have implications for access and integrity (both of which are outside the scope of this report), and states

---

2 Kavanagh et al., 2020.

must consider current laws and logistical considerations as well before pursuing such a change.[3] It is also relevant that we found only moderate levels of support among respondents for further expansion of mail-in options, such as sending a mail ballot to all registered voters whether they requested it or not, and very little support for more-dramatic shifts, such as one to online voting (perhaps because of greater security concerns with these options). This suggests that state and local officials might consider mitigating safety concerns with relatively modest changes to processes (such as eliminating the excuse requirement for mail-in voting) and might not need more-significant changes that have modest or low support. There will not be one approach that works everywhere, but the analysis here can be one factor among many informing policymaker choices.

Messaging Targeted at Groups That Question Safety, Integrity, and Preparedness Might Be Most Efficient at Mitigating Voter Concerns

Our analyses clearly showed that different groups have different perceptions of safety, election integrity, and preparedness of local officials for the 2020 election and that these perceptions have different effects on respondents' intention to vote. Although election officials and policymakers might wish to communicate broadly about their preparations for the 2020 election, our analyses suggest that such a campaign's effects would be maximized by targeting these messages at specific groups that seem most prone to such concerns. First, younger voters seem to have more concerns than do older voters, but older respondents appear to be more influenced by any negative perceptions when choosing whether to vote. In this case, messages might need to be developed for each audience. Second, minority groups appear to be more likely to have concerns about safety, election integrity, and preparedness. Notably, young and minority voters generally tend to have lower turnout rates than relevant comparison groups.[4] For policymakers interested in ensuring that the pandemic does not drive further disparities in

[3] Hodgson et al., 2020.

[4] Jens Manuel Krogstad, Luis Noe-Bustamante, and Antonio Flores, "Historic Highs in 2018 Voter Turnout Extended Across Racial and Ethnic Groups," Pew Research Center, May 1, 2019.

this area, targeted communication to these groups could be a useful tool. Finally, we note that Republican and Democratic respondents appeared to differ in their perceptions of risk: Republicans expressed more concern about election integrity; Democrats expressed more concern about safety. This reaffirms the notion that any communication strategy must equally emphasize both dimensions.

Final Thoughts

Efforts to understand how voters perceive the public health and election integrity risks stemming from the pandemic and how such risks might affect voting behavior will be ongoing between now and the November election. The trajectory of the pandemic, individual risk tolerance, mitigation strategies and messaging campaigns by election officials, and the changing political and social context are all likely to inform individuals' perceptions and intention to vote.

This report provides a baseline for exploring the evolution of these attitudes over the next several months, and the insights provided herein can inform policymakers and election officials who have an interest in mitigating voter safety and integrity concerns. However, a few caveats—also noted elsewhere in the report—are worth discussing here. First, when assessing expectations about safety and integrity, we cannot determine the extent to which an individual's response is based on assumptions about mitigations that public officials will take or about the trajectory of the virus. If such assumptions are factored in, then individual expectations might look very different. Second, when comparing intention to vote among 2016 respondents with that of 2020 respondents, we can only say that, in general, we saw no dramatic change. We cannot directly attribute this to a lack of response to the pandemic because any individual's decision to vote is based on myriad considerations. An individual might be substantially negatively influenced by the pandemic in their intention to vote but be positively influenced to the same degree by the political context or a desire to vote for a specific candidate.

Finally, our survey results—and, by extension, the results of our analysis—are likely influenced by the point in time at which the survey was conducted. Late May and early June was a period during which the most-severe effects of the pandemic had been felt in the Northeast and mid-Atlantic region, when the majority of states in this region turned the corner and were approaching reopening. Two months later, the picture already looks different, with the virus having surged in the South and the West and with some states reinstituting restrictions.[5] These are changes that could have effects on public attitudes.

There will likely be many more changes that might influence voter attitudes about the safety of the election and their intention to vote. Similarly, attitudes about election integrity might also evolve, depending on primary election experiences or steps taken by local officials (to the extent that this occurs). Continuing to track voter attitudes about the 2020 general election, their perceptions of safety and integrity, and their intention to vote through the fall (along with a post-election survey to assess outcomes) will be important for two reasons. First, doing so can continue to inform policymakers' and election officials' mitigation and messaging efforts. Second, continued tracking can contribute to our understanding of factors that influence intention to vote, both generally and in extraordinary circumstances, such as the current one.

---

[5] Randy Yeip, "How the COVID-19 Surge Shifted to the South and the West," *Wall Street Journal*, July 3, 2020.

APPENDIX

Weighted Characteristics and Regression Models

We surveyed 2,389 people using a nationally representative sample originally selected for RAND's American Life Panel (ALP). Respondents who had previously reported their demographics for the ALP were given an online survey of additional questions related to their previous voting behavior, future expected voting behavior, and attitudes regarding the election. Specifically, the questions asked were as follows:

- When was the last time you voted in any national/state/local election? How did you cast your ballot?[1]
- What is the percent chance that you will vote in the 2020 presidential election?
- Assuming you do vote, how do you expect to cast your ballot?[2]
- Assuming you do vote, when you think about voting in November 2020, do you feel that you will be safe from risks to your physical health stemming from COVID-19? (response options: yes, no, unsure)
- Assuming that you do vote, do you feel that your vote will be counted accurately in light of the current pandemic? (response options: yes, no, unsure)

---

1 Response options were: in person at a polling place, requested and returned an absentee ballot because I could not vote in person on Election Day, voted by mail (returned ballot by postal service), voted by mail (returned ballot to polling place or to local registrar's office).

2 Response options were: in person at a polling place, will request and return an absentee ballot because I cannot vote in person on Election Day, vote by mail (return ballot by postal service), vote by mail (return ballot to polling place or to local registrar's office).

- Do you believe your local elections officials are prepared to safeguard your physical health from risks associated with COVID-19 during the 2020 presidential election? (response options: yes, no, unsure)
- What measures do you think elections officials should take to safeguard your physical health from risks associated with COVID-19 during the 2020 presidential election? (Three options were provided; respondents could check all that applied: sanitation and social distancing; send mail-in ballots to all registered voters; online voting)

Table A.1 summarizes the weighted demographic characteristics of our sample. Our sample featured somewhat more men than women, was 69.7 percent White/Caucasian and 15.6 percent Black/African American, based on self-identified demographic information. About 22 percent of respondents were Hispanic. A little more than 20 percent lived in rural communities of less than 50,000 people; the rest lived in bigger cities. In these counts and in other percentages reported already, we used weights that adjust for partisanship and voting history, in addition to other demographic characteristics.

We also used data on whether respondents' states allowed mail-in voting without an excuse, drawing from RAND-collected data on state-level voting policies for the 2020 U.S. election. States were divided into two groups: those that allowed mail-in ballots only with an excuse and those that had some universal mail-in option. Many respondents did not report their state of residence, however, resulting in 380 missing values.

Perceptions of Safety, Election Integrity, and Preparedness

Regression models were used to model self-reported perceptions of safety, election integrity, and preparedness, as well as intention to vote. We measured those terms as follows:

Table A.1
Demographics of Omnibus Sample

Characteristic	Female	Male	Totals
Total	1,261 (52.8%)	1,128 (47.2%)	2,389
Race			
White/Caucasian	905 (71.8%)	760 (67.3%)	1,665 (69.7%)
American Indian or Alaska Native	59 (4.7%)	8 (0.7%)	67 (2.8%)
Asian or Pacific Islander	39 (3.1%)	39 (3.5%)	78 (3.3%)
Black/African American	178 (14.1%)	195 (17.3%)	373 (15.6%)
Other	80 (6.3%)	127 (11.2%)	207 (8.7%)
Ethnicity			
Non-Hispanic	965 (76.6%)	903 (80.0%)	1,868 (78.2%)
Hispanic	295 (23.4%)	226 (20.0%)	521 (21.8%)
Mean age (standard deviation)	50 (14)	49 (13)	50 (0)
Rural/urban status			
Population under 50,000	278 (22.1%)	217 (19.3%)	495 (20.8%)
Population over 50,000	978 (77.9%)	910 (80.7%)	1,888 (79.2%)

- *Safety* was measured using the question "Do you feel that you will be safe from risks to your physical health stemming from COVID-19?"
- *Election integrity* was measured using the question "Do you feel that your vote will be counted accurately in light of the current pandemic?"
- *Preparedness* was measured using the question "Do you believe your local elections officials are prepared to safeguard your physical health from risks associated with COVID-19 during the 2020 presidential election?"

For each of these questions, we reduced the responses to dummy variables, where 1 = "yes" and 0 = "no" or "not sure" for each measure.

We then applied logistic regression to predict whether respondents would answer "yes" to each question, respectively. A nearly identical formula was used to model each question, using geographic, demographic, and political preference characteristics as predictors. We considered two models, one without interaction effects and one in which we interacted each of these variables with perceptions of safety, election integrity, and preparedness. We used the interactions to determine whether partisanship, demographics, or geographic location had differing effects on the relationships between perception variables. For example, respondents in states with more access to mail-in voting options might not make as strong of a connection between perceptions of safety and election integrity compared with those who do not have those options. However, in general, the key results were the same across models, and the inclusion of interaction terms did not yield significant additional insights.

To ensure that models were not overspecified or affected by the number of variables, we compared the main effects in both models. We expected that respondents' views of the connections among safety, election integrity, and preparedness would differ according to political preferences, region of residence, and demographics. All models were selected using stepwise Akaike information criterion (AIC) selection. AIC is a measure of out-of-sample prediction error equal to the remaining unexplained deviance of the dependent variable plus a penalty for the number of variables used in the model. AIC is a standard measure of overall fit analogous to R-squared in linear regression. Tables A.2 through A.4 show these results. The model in Table A.4 serves as a robustness check to assess whether the inclusion of all perception variables in all models might cause issues of multicollinearity. Although we expected high potential of multicollinearity among perceptions of integrity, preparedness, and safety, the correlations between these values did not exceed 0.41; we also tried models with a combined measure summing all three into a 0–3 measure, with 0 meaning responding "yes" to none of the three questions, and 3 meaning that the respondent responded "yes" to all three survey questions. Model fit was better when examining the three variables separately. The model in Table A.4

considers only one perception variable at a time, but we found that the results are largely the same as the combined model.

Education was combined into three bins: less than a college degree, college degree, and postgraduate degree. This configuration was chosen to aggregate respondents into larger categories and enable us to estimate interaction effects, and it had better model fit than other configurations.

Past voting behavior was constructed using a fill-in box under the question, "When was the last time you voted in any national/state/local election?" The fill-in box asked for a year, but many respondents instead put "four years ago," a month and year in digit form (e.g., "11/16"), or other answers (e.g., "all of them"). However, all cases of a nonstandard answer were unambiguous and the intended meaning was clear in every case. We coded those who voted in 2016 or beyond as 1 and coded those who did not as 0. Respondents were also given the opportunity to check "not sure/don't remember" or "don't usually vote," which were both coded as 0. Although weights were not used in these models because of a lack of principled methodology for model selection using weighted regression, we did use weights in the predicted probabilities for these and other regression models to better reflect population percentages. We also explored the use of similar weighted models for the sake of comparison. Weighted and unweighted models were not substantially different.

Mitigation Preferences

We used logistic regression to predict support for potential election safeguards from COVID-19. We asked respondents whether they supported three mitigation measures: social-distancing measures for in-person voting, mail-in voting, and online voting. Responses were not exclusive, and respondents could show support for just one or all of the potential safeguards. Separate logistic regression models were applied to each safeguard, each with demographic, geographic, and political preference characteristics serving as predictors. The results are shown in Table A.5.

Table A.2
Logistic Regression Models Predicting Positive Perceptions of Safety, Election Integrity, and Preparedness

Effect	Safety	Integrity	Preparedness
(Intercept)	−0.93 (0.5)	−2.57 (0.52)***	−1.84 (0.49)***
Age (sq rt)	−0.09 (0.06)	0.19 (0.06)**	0.2 (0.06)***
Political affiliation (compared with Democrat)			
Independent	0.57 (0.15)***	−0.07 (0.15)	−0.29 (0.14)*
Not sure	0 (0.24)	−0.48 (0.24)	−0.31 (0.24)
Other	0.81 (0.28)**	−0.57 (0.26)*	−0.28 (0.26)
Republican	1.44 (0.16)***	−0.48 (0.15)**	0.33 (0.15)*
Male (compared with female)	0.24 (0.12)*	0.53 (0.11)***	−0.25 (0.11)*
Education (compared with less than a college degree)			
College degree		0.25 (0.13)	−0.01 (0.13)
Postgraduate degree		0.55 (0.15)***	−0.33 (0.15)*
Perception of safety *Response to: Do you feel that you will be safe from risks to your physical health stemming from COVID-19?*		0.59 (0.12)***	1.48 (0.12)***
Perception of election integrity *Response to: Do you feel that your vote will be counted accurately in light of the current pandemic?*	0.57 (0.12)***		1.13 (0.12)***
Perception of preparedness *Response to: Do you believe local elections officials are prepared to safeguard your physical health from risks associated with COVID-19 during the 2020 presidential election?*	1.47 (0.12)***	1.12 (0.12)***	

Table A.2—Continued

Effect	Safety	Integrity	Preparedness
Voted in 2016 and/or 2018	0.63 (0.16)***	0.46 (0.16)**	
Last reported vote method (compared with in person)			
Other	–1.73 (0.4)***		–0.91 (0.36)*
Requested and/or returned an absentee ballot	–0.23 (0.23)		–0.52 (0.23)*
Voted by mail (in person)	–0.01 (0.23)		–0.31 (0.21)
Voted by mail (post)	–0.18 (0.14)		–0.57 (0.13)***
Region (compared with Northeast)			
Midwest	–0.02 (0.19)	0.63 (0.18)***	
South	–0.11 (0.16)	0.29 (0.15)	
West	0.57 (0.2)**	0.22 (0.16)	
Hispanic ethnicity		–0.49 (0.19)**	
Race (compared with White/ Caucasian)			
American Indian or Alaska Native		–0.41 (0.53)	
Asian or Pacific Islander		0.58 (0.34)	
Black/African American		–0.67 (0.2)***	
Other		–0.13 (0.25)	
Urban (compared with rural)			–0.4 (0.14)**
No-excuse vote-by-mail option in state	–0.25 (0.14)		
Null deviance	2,466	2,429	2,518
AIC	1,968	2,082	2,051
N	1,912	1,912	1,912

* $p < 0.05$, ** $p < 0.01$, *** $p < 0.001$.

Table A.3
Logistic Regression Models Predicting Positive Perceptions of Safety, Election Integrity, and Local Official Preparedness with Interactions

Effect	Safety	Integrity	Preparedness
(Intercept)	–0.94 (0.53)	–2.79 (0.55)***	–1.87 (0.53)***
Age (sq rt)	–0.1 (0.06)	0.21 (0.06)***	0.21 (0.06)***
Education (compared with less than a college degree)			
College degree	0.16 (0.24)	0.23 (0.13)	–0.34 (0.21)
Postgraduate degree	–0.27 (0.28)	0.54 (0.15)***	–0.43 (0.23)
Political affiliation (compared with Democrat)			
Independent	0.55 (0.15)***	0.08 (0.23)	–0.29 (0.15)*
Not sure	–0.06 (0.25)	–0.31 (0.33)	–0.38 (0.24)
Other	0.83 (0.28)**	–1.09 (0.48)*	–0.31 (0.26)
Republican	1.42 (0.16)***	0.21 (0.28)	0.33 (0.15)*
Last reported vote method (compared with in person)			
Other	–1.2 (0.52)*	–0.47 (0.46)	–0.9 (0.36)*
Requested and/or returned an absentee ballot	0.42 (0.37)	–0.17 (0.41)	–0.52 (0.23)*
Voted by mail (in person)	–0.25 (0.38)	0.07 (0.45)	–0.35 (0.21)
Voted by mail (post)	–0.37 (0.22)	0.29 (0.25)	–0.58 (0.13)***
Male	0.58 (0.2)**	0.75 (0.23)***	–0.25 (0.11)*
Hispanic ethnicity		–0.46 (0.2)*	0.44 (0.25)
Perception of safety *Response to: Do you feel that you will be safe from risks to your physical health stemming from COVID-19?*		0.55 (0.32)	1.29 (0.21)***
Perception of election integrity *Response to: Do you feel that your vote will be counted accurately in light of the current pandemic?*	1.03 (0.24)***		1.16 (0.12)***

Table A.3—Continued

Effect	Safety	Integrity	Preparedness
Perception of preparedness *Response to: Do you believe local elections officials are prepared to safeguard your physical health from risks associated with COVID-19 during the 2020 presidential election?*	1.14 (0.2)***	0.6 (0.29)*	
Voted in 2016 and/or 2018	0.62 (0.16)***	0.44 (0.16)**	
Region (compared with Northeast)			
Midwest	0 (0.19)	0.66 (0.19)***	
South	−0.09 (0.16)	0.28 (0.16)	
West	0.62 (0.2)**	0.12 (0.18)	
Perception of safety * education			
College degree			0.58 (0.27)*
Postgraduate degree			0.22 (0.29)
Perception of safety * Hispanic ethnicity			−0.57 (0.33)
Perception of safety * political affiliation			
Independent		−0.33 (0.31)	
Not sure		−0.38 (0.48)	
Other		0.76 (0.59)	
Perception of integrity * education			
College degree	−0.68 (0.28)*		
Postgraduate degree	−0.12 (0.32)		
Perception of integrity * last reported vote method			
Other	−1.18 (0.79)		

Table A.3—Continued

Effect	Safety	Integrity	Preparedness
Requested and/or returned an absentee ballot	−0.96 (0.47)*		
Voted by mail (in person)	0.39 (0.47)		
Voted by mail (post)	0.24 (0.27)		
Perception of integrity * male	−0.47 (0.25)		
Perception of preparedness * education			
College degree	0.6 (0.28)*		
Postgraduate degree	0.4 (0.3)		
Perception of preparedness * last reported vote method			
Other		0.71 (1.04)	
Voted using absentee ballot		1.9 (0.97)	
Voted by mail (in person)		0.37 (0.75)	
Voted by mail (post)		−0.29 (0.42)	
Perception of preparedness * male		0.31 (0.4)	
Race (compared with White/ Caucasian)			
American Indian or Alaska Native		−0.59 (0.56)	
Asian or Pacific Islander		0.57 (0.35)	
Black/African American		−0.66 (0.21)**	
Other		−0.16 (0.25)	
Perception of preparedness * last reported vote method			
Other		0.45 (1.34)	

Table A.3—Continued

Effect	Safety	Integrity	Preparedness
Requested and/or returned an absentee ballot		−0.26 (0.65)	
Voted by mail (in person)		0.84 (0.67)	
Voted by mail (post)		−0.28 (0.38)	
Perception of preparedness * perception of safety		1.01 (0.39)*	
Perception of preparedness * perception of safety * last reported vote method			
Other		−1.99 (1.81)	
Requested and/or returned an absentee ballot		−1.94 (1.16)	
Voted by mail (in person)		−1.69 (0.95)	
Voted by mail (post)		0.83 (0.56)	
Perception of preparedness * perception of safety * male		−0.73 (0.5)	
Perception of safety * male		−0.13 (0.34)	
Urban (compared with rural)			−0.42 (0.14)**
No-excuse vote-by-mail option in state	−0.24 (0.14)		
Null deviance	2,466	2,429	2,518
AIC	1,965	2,076	2,049
N	1,912	1,912	1,912

* $p < 0.05$, ** $p < 0.01$, *** $p < 0.001$.

Table A.4
Logistic Regression Models Predicting Positive Perceptions of Safety, Election Integrity, and Preparedness, Robustness Checks

Effect	Safety	Integrity	Preparedness
Intercept	−0.59 (0.19)**	−2.3 (0.48)***	−1.28 (0.46)**
Age (sq rt)		0.25 (0.06)***	0.24 (0.06)***
Voted in 2016 and/or 2018	0.79 (0.15)***	0.72 (0.14)***	0.48 (0.15)***
Last reported vote method (compared with in person)			
Other	−2.1 (0.38)***	−1.05 (0.32)***	−1.58 (0.33)***
Requested and/or returned an absentee ballot	−0.43 (0.21)*	−0.32 (0.22)	−0.65 (0.21)**
Voted by mail (in person)	−0.1 (0.22)	−0.06 (0.21)	−0.38 (0.2)
Voted by mail (post)	−0.32 (0.13)*	0.06 (0.13)	−0.6 (0.13)***
Region (compared with Northeast)			
Midwest	0.2 (0.17)	0.63 (0.18)***	0.17 (0.17)
South	−0.1 (0.15)	0.21 (0.15)	−0.16 (0.14)
West	0.79 (0.17)***	0.27 (0.16)	0.35 (0.16)*
Education (compared with less than a college degree)			
College degree		0.28 (0.12)*	0.1 (0.12)
Postgraduate degree		0.45 (0.14)**	−0.2 (0.13)
Hispanic ethnicity	−0.31 (0.16)	−0.52 (0.18)**	
Political affiliation (compared with Democrat)			
Independent	0.47 (0.14)***		−0.07 (0.13)
Not sure	−0.15 (0.23)		−0.42 (0.22)
Other	0.62 (0.26)*		−0.1 (0.24)
Republican	1.52 (0.15)***		0.72 (0.14)***

Table A.4—Continued

Effect	Safety	Integrity	Preparedness
Voted in 2016 and/or 2018	0.27 (0.11)*	0.51 (0.11)***	
Race (compared with White/ Caucasian)			
American Indian or Alaska Native		−0.55 (0.52)	
Asian or Pacific Islander		0.39 (0.33)	
Black/African American		−0.67 (0.18)***	
Other		−0.17 (0.23)	
Urban (compared with rural)			−0.4 (0.13)**
Null deviance	2,466	2,429	2,518
AIC	2,187	2,234	2,340
N	1,912	1,912	1,912

* $p < 0.05$, ** $p < 0.01$, *** $p < 0.001$.

Voting Intentions

We also asked respondents, "What is the percent chance that you will vote in the 2020 presidential election?" with a slider bar that respondents manipulated with their mouse. We added a qualifier below the question, "The percent chance can be thought of as the number of chances out of 100. You can use any number between 0 and 100. For example, numbers like 2 and 5 percent might be 'almost no chance,' 20 percent or so might mean 'not much chance,' a 45- or 55-percent chance might be a 'pretty even chance,' 80 percent or so might mean a 'very good chance,' and a 95- or 98-percent chance might be 'almost certain.'" The respondents were most likely to move the indicator near the right side to indicate a certain or near-certain probability that they would vote. The next most-common ranges were a middle group (around 50) and a low-end group (about 0–10), each seemingly with its own distribution. Because the dependent variable was not normally distributed, we decided against a linear model and instead divided

Table A.5
Logistic Regression of Mitigation Preferences

Effect	Social Distancing	Universal Mail-In	Online Voting
Intercept	2.98 (0.58)***	1.06 (0.22)***	2.28 (0.48)***
Political affiliation (compared with Democrat)			
Independent	−0.01 (0.16)	−1.24 (0.14)***	−0.24 (0.13)
Not sure	−0.36 (0.24)	−1.41 (0.22)***	−0.03 (0.21)
Other	−0.15 (0.28)	−1.66 (0.25)***	−0.24 (0.24)
Republican	0.98 (0.18)***	−2.89 (0.15)***	−1.04 (0.14)***
Region (compared with Northeast)			
Midwest	−0.37 (0.22)	−0.18 (0.19)	−0.43 (0.18)*
South	−0.2 (0.2)	−0.24 (0.16)	−0.06 (0.14)
West	−0.86 (0.19)***	0.6 (0.19)**	−0.64 (0.17)***
Age (sq rt)	−0.18 (0.07)*		−0.35 (0.06)***
Education (compared with less than a college degree)			
College degree	0.28 (0.14)	0.19 (0.13)	
Postgraduate degree	0.42 (0.17)*	0.4 (0.15)**	
Hispanic ethnicity		−0.44 (0.19)*	0.37 (0.16)*
Urban (compared with rural)		0.55 (0.14)***	0.5 (0.14)***
No-excuse vote-by-mail option in state		−0.55 (0.14)***	−0.24 (0.13)
Race (compared with White/Caucasian)			
American Indian or Alaska Native		0.77 (0.6)	
Asian or Pacific Islander		0.35 (0.34)	
Black/African American		−0.47 (0.2)*	
Other		−0.39 (0.25)	
Male			−0.32 (0.11)**
Null deviance	1,743	2,638	2,434
AIC	1,678	2,049	2,258
N	1,912	1,912	1,912

* $p < 0.05$, ** $p < 0.01$, *** $p < 0.001$.

the responses into three categories according to these three observed clusters of responses. We divided the answers according to each range: very low probability of voting in 2020 (< 35 percent chance), mixed or unsure (35- to 75-percent chance), and certain or almost certain (> 75 percent). We then applied ordinal logistic regression to the results to predict respondents' membership in each group by demographic and geographic characteristics (with a categorical variable for U.S. region) and attitudes regarding safety, election integrity, and preparedness.

The initial model formula interacted past voting behavior with all other variables because we expected that those groups could be considered separately in their future intention. We also interacted perceptions of safety, election integrity, and preparedness with demographic, geographic, and political preference variables because we expected that these perceptions would be associated with intention to vote in different ways for different categories of respondents. For example, groups known to be more likely to have preexisting health issues (e.g., older respondents, Black/African American respondents) might be more hesitant to vote if they perceive the election to be unsafe as a result of COVID-19. For all models, we used AIC for stepwise model selection, discarding variables that did not independently contribute to lower AIC values. To ensure that the model was not overspecified and was not influenced by the number of variables, we also ran a model without interactions and found that the main effects were unchanged by the inclusion of additional variables. Table A.6 reports the results of the final model. Table A.7 acts as a check on multicollinearity among the three perception variables, and each model features only one of the three variables. We found that the results are largely the same, whether each perception is examined separately or they are all grouped together.

Separately, we ran a similar model looking specifically at the impact of past intention to vote on future intention to vote. We specified a model with all variables interacted with the intention to vote measured in 2016. The model is specified without any additional three-way interactions to preserve power. The results are shown in Table A.8.

A final set of models explored what factors led to respondents intending to switch from voting in person to a remote method. These models considered only those respondents who voted in person as their

Table A.6
Ordered Logistic Regression of Intention to Vote

Effect	Coefficient (standard error)
Perception of safety *Response to: Do you feel that you will be safe from risks to your physical health stemming from COVID-19?*	0.93 (0.25)***
Perception of integrity *Response to: Do you feel that your vote will be counted accurately in light of the current pandemic?*	0.71 (0.29)*
Voted in 2016 and/or 2018	3.26 (0.21)***
Race (compared with White/Caucasian)	
American Indian or Alaska Native	0.62 (0.82)
Asian or Pacific Islander	–1.43 (0.65)*
Black/African American	0.52 (0.41)
Other	0.33 (0.41)
Urban (compared with rural)	–0.51 (0.29)
Education (compared with less than a college degree)	
College degree	0.66 (0.31)*
Postgraduate degree	1.39 (0.47)**
Political affiliation (compared with Democrat)	
Republican	–0.04 (0.32)
Independent	–0.59 (0.27)*
Other	–1.83 (0.36)***
Not sure	–1.29 (0.29)***
Hispanic ethnicity	–0.46 (0.25)
Perception of safety * race	
American Indian or Alaska Native	–2.14 (1.27)
Asian or Pacific Islander	1.73 (1.06)
Black/African American	–1.29 (0.58)*
Other	–1.2 (0.56)*

Table A.6—Continued

Effect	Coefficient (standard error)
Perception of integrity * education	
College degree	−0.53 (0.44)
Postgraduate degree	−1.31 (0.61)*
1|2[a]	−1.1 (0.4)**
2|3[b]	−0.04 (0.39)
Null deviance	1,579
Residual deviance	941
N	1,901

* $p < 0.05$, ** $p < 0.01$, *** $p < 0.001$.

[a] 1|2 is the logged odds of being in category 1 versus 2 or 3.

[b] 2|3 is the logged odds of being in category 1 or 2 compared with 3, where categories refer to certain not to vote, uncertain to vote, and certain to vote.

latest voting method and were coded as 1 if they intended on switching in 2020. We used whether they voted in 2016 or 2018; perceptions of integrity, safety, and preparedness; and demographic, geographic, and political preference characteristics as independent variables. The results are shown in Table A.9.

Table A.7
Ordered Logistic Regression of Intention to Vote, Robustness Checks

Effect	Safety Perception Only	Legitimacy Perception Only	Preparedness Perception Only	Full Model
Education (compared with less than a college degree)				
College degree	0.39 (0.21)	0.42 (0.21)	0.43 (0.21)*	0.39 (0.21)
Postgraduate degree	0.6 (0.29)*	0.56 (0.29)	0.58 (0.29)*	0.6 (0.29)*
Hispanic ethnicity	−0.53 (0.23)*	−0.53 (0.23)*	−0.56 (0.23)*	−0.53 (0.23)*
Political affiliation (compared with Democrat)				
Independent	−0.55 (0.26)*	−0.46 (0.26)	−0.5 (0.26)	−0.55 (0.26)*
Not sure	−1.36 (0.28)***	−1.34 (0.28)***	−1.4 (0.28)***	−1.36 (0.28)***
Other	−1.92 (0.35)***	−1.8 (0.34)***	−1.87 (0.34)***	−1.92 (0.35)***
Republican	0.09 (0.31)	0.26 (0.3)	0.26 (0.3)	0.09 (0.31)
Voted in 2016 and/or 2018	3.25 (0.21)***	3.27 (0.21)***	3.32 (0.21)***	3.25 (0.21)***
Perception of safety *Response to: Do you feel that you will be safe from risks to your physical health stemming from COVID-19?*	0.7 (0.2)***			0.7 (0.2)***

Table A.7—Continued

Effect	Safety Perception Only	Legitimacy Perception Only	Preparedness Perception Only	Full Model
Perception of election integrity *Response to: Do you feel that your vote will be counted accurately in light of the current pandemic?*		0.38 (0.2)		
Perception of preparedness *Response to: Do you believe local elections officials are prepared to safeguard your physical health from risks associated with COVID-19 during the 2020 presidential election?*				
Male (compared with female)			0.29 (0.2)	
Urban (compared with rural)	−0.58 (0.28)*	−0.55 (0.28)	−0.55 (0.28)*	−0.58 (0.28)*
Null deviance	1,579	1,579	1,579	1,579
Residual deviance	963	972	974	963
1|2[a]	−1.53 (0.36)***	−1.58 (0.36 ***	−1.66 (0.35)***	−1.53 (0.36)***
2|3[b]	−0.51 (0.35)	−0.57 (0.36)	−0.67 (0.35)	−0.51 (0.35)
N	1,901	1,901	1,901	1,901

* $p < 0.05$, ** $p < 0.01$, *** $p < 0.001$.

[a] 1|2 is the logged odds of being in category 1 versus 2 or 3.

[b] 2|3 is the logged odds of being in category 1 or 2 compared with 3, where categories refer to certain not to vote, uncertain to vote, and certain to vote.

Table A.8
Ordered Logistic Regression Models, Past Intention on Future Intention to Vote

Effect	Coefficient (standard error)
2016 reported voting chance	−0.01 (0.01)
Perception of safety *Response to: Do you feel that you will be safe from risks to your physical health stemming from COVID-19?*	0.46 (0.28)
Perception of integrity *Response to: Do you feel that your vote will be counted accurately in light of the current pandemic?*	0.77 (0.47)
Perception of preparedness *Response to: Do you believe local elections officials are prepared to safeguard your physical health from risks associated with COVID-19 during the 2020 presidential election?*	1.81 (0.49)***
Age (sq rt)	−0.58 (0.09)***
Urban (compared with rural)	−0.93 (0.39)*
Education (compared with less than a college degree)	
College degree	0.57 (0.28)*
Postgraduate degree	1.42 (0.42)***
Vote-by-mail option in state	−0.11 (0.54)
Political affiliation (compared with Democrat)	
Republican	−0.08 (0.39)
Independent	−0.43 (0.35)
Other	−1.66 (0.49)***
Not sure	−1.55 (0.38)***
Region (compared with Northeast)	
South	1.24 (0.36)***
Midwest	0.05 (0.44)
West	0.24 (0.43)
Hispanic ethnicity	0.18 (0.54)

Table A.8—Continued

Effect	Coefficient (standard error)
2016 reported voting chance * perception of preparedness	−0.02 (0.01)*
2016 reported voting chance * perception of integrity	−0.01 (0.01)
2016 reported voting chance * age (sq rt)	0.01 (0.00)***
2016 reported voting chance * vote-by-mail option in state	−0.01 (0.01)
2016 reported voting chance * Hispanic ethnicity	−0.02 (0.01)**
1|2[a]	−3.03 (0.08)***
2|3[b]	−1.57 (0.18)***
Null deviance	1,135
Residual deviance	579
N	1,589

* $p < 0.05$, ** $p < 0.01$, *** $p < 0.001$.

[a] 1|2 is the logged odds of being in category 1 versus 2 or 3.

[b] 2|3 is the logged odds of being in category 1 or 2 compared with 3, where categories refer to certain not to vote, uncertain to vote, and certain to vote.

Table A.9
Logistic Regression Models Predicting Switching from In-Person to Remote Voting with Interactions

Effect	Coefficient (standard error)
Intercept	–1.02 (0.37)**
Perception of safety *Response to: Do you feel that you will be safe from risks to your physical health stemming from COVID-19?*	0.92 (0.43)*
Urban (compared with rural)	0.83 (0.32)**
Vote-by-mail option in state	–0.21 (0.23)
Political affiliation (compared with Democrat)	
Republican	–0.95 (0.39)*
Independent	0.03 (0.26)
Other	1.03 (0.72)
Not sure	0.01 (0.64)
Region (compared with Northeast)	
South	–0.13 (0.2)
Midwest	–0.33 (0.25)
West	0.61 (0.26)*
Perception of safety * urban	–0.88 (0.41)*
Perception of safety * vote-by-mail option in state	–0.99 (0.34)**
Perception of safety * political affiliation (compared with Democrat)	
Republican	–1.35 (0.48)**
Independent	–1.00 (0.37)**
Other	–2.72 (0.96)**
Not sure	–1.11 (0.92)
Null deviance	1,250
Residual deviance	1,078
N	1,127

* $p < 0.05$, ** $p < 0.01$, *** $p < 0.001$.

References

Achen, Christopher H., and André Blais, "Intention to Vote, Reported Vote, and Validated Vote," in Johan A. Elkink and David M. Farrell, eds., *The Act of Voting: Identities, Institutions and Locale*, London: Routledge, 2015, pp. 195–209.

Ajzen, Icek, "From Intentions to Actions: A Theory of Planned Behavior," in Julius Kuhl and Jürgen Beckmann, eds., *Action Control: From Cognition to Behavior*, Berlin: Springer, 1985, pp. 11–39.

Berinsky, Adam J., Nancy Burns, and Michael W. Traugott, "Who Votes by Mail? A Dynamic Model of the Individual-Level Consequences of Voting-by-Mail Systems," *Public Opinion Quarterly*, Vol. 65, No. 2, 2001, pp. 178–197.

Birch, Sarah, "Perceptions of Electoral Fairness and Voter Turnout," *Comparative Political Studies*, Vol. 43, No. 12, 2010, pp. 1601–1622.

Brehm, John O., *The Phantom Respondents: Opinion Surveys and Political Representation*, Ann Arbor: University of Michigan Press, 2009.

Carreras, Miguel, and Yasemin İrepoğlu, "Trust in Elections, Vote Buying, and Turnout in Latin America," *Electoral Studies*, Vol. 32, No. 4, 2013, pp. 609–619.

Collier, Paul, and Pedro C. Vicente, "Votes and Violence: Evidence from a Field Experiment in Nigeria," *Economic Journal*, Vol. 124, No. 574, 2014, pp. F327–F355.

Dalton, Russell J., "The Social Transformation of Trust in Government," *International Review of Sociology*, Vol. 15, No. 1, 2005, pp. 133–154.

Darmofal, David, "Elite Cues and Citizen Disagreement with Expert Opinion," *Political Research Quarterly*, Vol. 58, No. 3, 2005, pp. 381–395.

Dubin, Jeffrey A., and Gretchen A. Kalsow, "Comparing Absentee and Precinct Voters: A View over Time," *Political Behavior*, Vol. 18, No. 4, 1996, pp. 369–392.

Glaser, William A., "Intention and Voting Turnout," *American Political Science Review*, Vol. 52, No. 4, 1958, pp. 1030–1040.

Granberg, Donald, and Soren Holmberg, "Self-Reported Turnout and Voter Validation," *American Journal of Political Science*, Vol. 35, No. 2, 1991, pp. 448–459.

Gregorian, Dareh, "Voter Turnout Soared in Georgia, Despite Massive Primary Day Problems," NBC News, June 12, 2020.

Hartig, Hannah, Bradley Jones, and Vianney Gomez, "As States Move to Expand the Practice, Relatively Few Americans Have Voted by Mail," Pew Research Center, June 24, 2020.

Hodgson, Quentin E., Jennifer Kavanagh, Anusree Garg, Edward W. Chan, and Christine Sovak, *Options for Ensuring Safe Elections: Preparing for Elections During a Pandemic*, Santa Monica, Calif.: RAND Corporation, RR-A112-10, 2020. As of August 5, 2020:
https://www.rand.org/pubs/research_reports/RRA112-10.html

Jones, Daniel B., Werner Troesken, and Randall Walsh, "Political Participation in a Violent Society: The Impact of Lynching on Voter Turnout in the Post-Reconstruction South," *Journal of Development Economics*, Vol. 129, 2017, pp. 29–46.

Kavanagh, Jennifer, Quentin E. Hodgson, C. Ben Gibson, and Samantha Cherney, *An Assessment of State Voting Processes: Preparing for Elections During a Pandemic*, Santa Monica, Calif.: RAND Corporation, RR-A112-8, 2020. As of August 5, 2020:
https://www.rand.org/pubs/research_reports/RRA112-8.html

Kavanagh, Jennifer, and Michael D. Rich, *Truth Decay: An Initial Exploration of the Diminishing Role of Facts and Analysis in American Public Life*, Santa Monica, Calif.: RAND Corporation, RR-2314-RC, 2018. As of August 2020:
https://www.rand.org/pubs/research_reports/RR2314.html

Koch, Jeffrey W., "Racial Minorities' Trust in Government and Government Decisionmakers," *Social Science Quarterly*, Vol. 100, No. 1, 2019, pp. 19–37.

Krogstad, Jens Manuel, Luis Noe-Bustamante, and Antonio Flores, "Historic Highs in 2018 Voter Turnout Extended Across Racial and Ethnic Groups," Pew Research Center, May 1, 2019.

Mallapaty, Smriti, "How Deadly Is the Coronavirus? Scientists Are Close to an Answer," *Nature*, Vol. 582, June 16, 2020, pp. 467–468.

Martinez i Coma, Ferran, and Minh Trinh, "How Electoral Integrity Affects Voter Turnout in Democracies," *Australian Journal of Political Science*, Vol. 52, No. 1, 2017, pp. 53–74.

Morris, Kevin, "Who Votes by Mail?" Brennan Center for Justice, April 15, 2020.

Pew Research Center, "Republicans, Democrats Move Even Further Apart in Coronavirus Concerns," June 25, 2020. As of July 31, 2020:
https://www.pewresearch.org/politics/2020/06/25/republicans-democrats-move-even-further-apart-in-coronavirus-concerns/

Pollard, Michael S., and Joshua Mendelsohn, *Methodology of the 2016 RAND Presidential Election Panel Survey (PEPS)*, RAND Corporation, RR-1460-RC/UCLA, 2016. As of July 29, 2020:
https://www.rand.org/pubs/research_reports/RR1460.html

Rainie, Lee, Scott Keeter, and Andrew Perrin, "Trust and Distrust in America," Pew Research Center, July 22, 2019. As of July 20, 2020:
https://www.pewresearch.org/politics/2019/07/22/trust-and-distrust-in-america/

RAND Corporation, "RAND American Life Panel," webpage, undated. As of July 27, 2020:
https://www.rand.org/research/data/alp.html

Southwell, Priscilla L., and Justin I. Burchett, "The Effect of All-Mail Elections on Voter Turnout," *American Politics Quarterly*, Vol. 28, No. 1, 2000, pp. 72–79.

Stewart, Charles III, "Election Updates: Mail Ballot Watch," MIT Election Data and Science Lab, July 6, 2020. As of July 20, 2020:
https://electionupdates.caltech.edu/2020/07/06/mail-ballot-watch/

Thompson, Daniel M., Jennifer Wu, Jesse Yoder, and Andrew B. Hall, *The Neutral Partisan Effects of Vote-by-Mail: Evidence from County-Level Roll-Outs*, Palo Alto, Calif.: Stanford Institute for Economic Policy Research, Working Paper 20-015, 2020a.

Thompson, Daniel M., Jennifer Wu, Jesse Yoder, and Andrew B. Hall, "Universal Vote-by-Mail Has No Impact on Partisan Turnout or Vote Share," *Proceedings of the National Academy of Sciences*, Vol. 117, No. 25, 2020b, pp. 14052–14056.

Trelles, Alejandro, and Miguel Carreras, "Bullets and Votes: Violence and Electoral Participation in Mexico," *Journal of Politics in Latin America*, Vol. 4, No. 2, 2012, pp. 89–123.

Ura, Alexa, "Two Major Texas Counties Are Trimming Polling Locations as Workers Pull Out over Coronavirus," *Texas Tribune*, July 9, 2020.

Wice, Sarah Ewall, "Kentucky on Track for Historic Turnout," CBS News, June 23, 2020.

Yeip, Randy, "How the COVID-19 Surge Shifted to the South and the West," *Wall Street Journal*, July 3, 2020.

About the Authors

Jennifer Kavanagh is a senior political scientist at the RAND Corporation and director of the Strategy, Doctrine, and Resources Program in the RAND Arroyo Center. She also leads RAND's Countering Truth Decay initiative, a portfolio of projects exploring the diminishing reliance on facts and analysis in U.S. political and civil discourse. Her research focuses on U.S. defense strategy, international conflict, disinformation, and the relationship between U.S. political and media institutions. She earned her Ph.D. in political science and public policy.

C. Ben Gibson is an associate behavioral/social scientist at the RAND Corporation. He has interests in conversation analysis, rumoring, information diffusion, and consensus formation; diffusion modeling in social networks; cybersecurity (both human factors and threat detection); statistical methodology, especially computational modeling of networks and other relational dynamics; informant accuracy and survey methods; and international conflict. He holds a Ph.D. in sociology.

Quentin E. Hodgson is a senior international and defense researcher at the RAND Corporation focusing on cybersecurity, cyber operations, critical infrastructure protection, risk management, and command and control. He has led projects for the U.S. Department of Defense, the U.S. Department of Homeland Security, and NATO's Allied Command Transformation. He holds an M.A. in international relations and an M.Sc. in national resource management, and was a Fulbright scholar affiliated with the University of Potsdam, Germany.